AF886467

Embrace Your Fertility

A Practical Guide to
Increasing Your Ability to Conceive

Timea Belej-Rak, M.D.

Fem Wellness

Copyright © 2022 Timea Belej-Rak, M.D.

All rights reserved. No part of this publication may be reproduced, distributed, or transmitted in any form or by any means, including photocopying, recording, or other electronic or mechanical methods without the prior written permission of the publisher.

This book is intended to provide general information only. Neither the author nor publisher provide any medical or other professional advice. If you need professional advice, you should seek advice from the appropriate licensed professional.

This book is intended to be used only as a general guide, and not as a sole source of information on the subject matter. The author and publisher shall have no liability or responsibility to any person or entity and hereby disclaim all liability, including without limitation, liability for consequential damages regarding any claim, loss or damage that may be incurred, or alleged to have been incurred, directly or indirectly, arising out of the information provided in this book.

Print Book ISBN: 978-1-990319-04-4

EBook ISBN: 978-1-990319-05-1

Shusia Publishing

This book is dedicated to all those who may be experiencing a fertility challenge.

May you find light and renewed hope in your fertility journey.

Embrace Your Fertility is a splendid book which covers everything you need to know and do to help you conceive a child or otherwise make peace with your fertility. It is written with the authoritative compassion of a physician who has not only been there herself, but has also helped hundreds of other individuals through the fertility journey. This book is a gem that I highly recommend to everyone who is concerned about her (or his) fertility."

Christiane Northrup, M.D., ob/gyn physician and author of the New York Times bestsellers: *Goddesses Never Age: The Secret Prescription for Radiance, Vitality, and Wellbeing; Women's Bodies, Women's Wisdom;* and *The Wisdom of Menopause*

Compiled by a spiritually-attuned, holistically conscious fertility specialist, **Embrace Your Fertility** is a comprehensive guide to navigating your fertility journey, complete with wisdom and knowledge about everything from conventional medical approaches to adoption to acupuncture to the mind-body perspectives that optimize fertility outcomes. Filled with stories of women who have navigated their own fertility experiences, readers will find comfort and inspiration alongside grounded, practical information.

Lissa Rankin, MD, New York Times bestselling author of *Mind Over Medicine*

Table of Contents

Foreword by Sara R. Cohen

Dear Readers,

It is my honor and pleasure to introduce to you, Embrace Your Fertility: Empowering You with Tools to Help You Succeed. I hope this book will be a meaningful journey for you, offering you the opportunity to look at your fertility struggle from new perspectives.

I am a fertility lawyer practicing exclusively in the area of fertility law, which typically includes third party reproduction (i.e. surrogacy, egg donation, sperm donation, embryo donation and the legal process whereby we make the intended parents the legal parents of the child). Some of my clients build their families through third party reproduction because they are struggling with infertility for a variety of reasons. Others use third party reproduction to conceive because they are single, or in a non-heteronormative relationship.

Whatever the reason, all people conceiving through assisted reproductive technologies have very important decisions to make that deal with extremely intimate parts of their lives. The more information, and the more options, the better. Embrace your Fertility looks at the fertility journey from many different perspectives and provides many different options. Not all will resonate with you, but certainly, many will.

Because of the confusing gray area brought into existence by the Assisted Human Reproduction Act, S.C. 2004, c.2, my endorsement of this book should not be seen as an endorsement of any business or activity contemplated in this book. However, I do hope you see it as an endorsement of some of the philosophies behind the book: that sometimes it takes a village and collaboration to build a family, that there are many different ways to build a family, and that there are many legitimate decisions and options that one could embrace at each turn. There is no right or wrong, and there is no straight path, but it is your path.

I received the invitation to introduce this book to you between two of the most significant dates of the fertility calendar. No, I am not referring to the date of ovulation or the two-week wait. I am referring to Mother's Day and Father's Day, a time often filled with pain for those trying to conceive.

Timea Belej-Rak, M.D.

If you are struggling with conception, I hope that you take comfort in the intimate stories shared by the prospective parents in this book. Even better, I hope that you find some of their stories inspiring. And I hope that you understand just how compassionate and empathetic are the doctors, counselors and other professionals involved in the fertility field. There is support available when you need it, other options to explore, and doors to open.

Most of all, I hope this book gives you hope.

Sincerely yours,

Sara R. Cohen, LL.B.

Fertility Law Canada Fellow, American Academy of Assisted Reproductive Technology Attorneys

www.fertilitylawcanada.com

Foreword by Janet Fraser

The inability to conceive and have the family that you have always dreamed of can be devastating and confusing. You may keep the issue to yourself, not wishing to share this information with your family and friends. That can make you feel lonely and unsure of where to turn for help. In addition, much of the published research is very clinical in nature and not easy to understand. This book is written to be a resource if you are having difficulty conceiving, providing straightforward information about the various options available.

As you read the book, you will discover that you are not alone. Each chapter starts with a potential parent's experience (in his or her own words) followed by a practitioner discussing how a particular treatment option can assist with conception from a physical, mental, and emotional perspective. The chapters are very informative, giving you a better understanding of how your body functions, what is required for you to be in optimal health, and how important a healthy body is when you are trying to conceive.

Unfortunately, not everyone who dreams of a family will be able to achieve it through natural means or by medical intervention. The last chapter discusses a different way to create your family—by adoption. It gives you an overview of some of the rules, regulations and hurdles that you may face, and it discusses the psychology of adopting.

I strongly believe that if you are experiencing fertility issues you should obtain as much information as possible to understand your options. I believe this book will help you achieve that goal.

Janet Fraser, BBA, MBA

President, Fertility Matters Canada

http://fertilitymatters.ca/

Acknowledgments

I am most grateful to the patients who chose to share their stories so that they could help you and others. Fertility issues are often experienced in isolation, and it is only through sharing our stories that we start letting the light shine through.

Some of our patients have expressed their wish to remain anonymous, and their names have been changed or removed from their stories. Others felt comfortable sharing their identities, and you can find out more about them in the contributor section at the back of the book.

I could not have done this project without the help of my co-authors, all of whom contributed their time, energy and wisdom, and to whom I will be forever grateful.

- A special thank you to our legal advisor Victoria Novak, who helped us understand what we were getting ourselves into.
- Thanks to our proof-reader Michelle Waitzman, for her eagle eye in picking up our discrepancies.
- I cannot thank our editor, Kathy Barthel, enough for her hard work and dedication to this project, which could not have been possible without her tireless efforts.
- Glenn Stewart Coles, thank you for rebranding our book and getting it ready for e-publishing and re-launch; your help and efforts are much appreciated!
- A special thank you to Sara Cohen and Janet Fraser for taking the time to read our manuscript and writing their forewords.
- A heartfelt thank you to Dr. Lissa Rankin and Dr. Christiane Northrup for their kind endorsements.

And finally, a big thank you to my family who supported me throughout this journey. I could not have done it without them!

It has been a pleasure and an honour to work with all of you!

Timea Belej-Rak, 2022

Introduction

Conception is such a mysterious, complex, and mind-blowing event that I fell in love with it in high school biology class. Cutting the cord of that first baby whose delivery I attended in medical school, solidified my belief that this was exactly what I wanted to do for the rest of my life. At first, it was delivering babies, however, once I discovered that I could actually play a role in creating them, there was no turning back! I have to thank my husband, who enabled me to complete my seventeen years of post-secondary education at the University of Toronto, for helping me to get the appropriate training for this journey. I am now thrilled to be able to share what I have learned over the past ten years with my patients, and those wishing to conceive.

Soon after I started practicing as a gynecologic reproductive endocrinologist and fertility specialist, I realized that many of my patients were also seeking help from other practitioners, such as acupuncturists, naturopaths and others. While our medical treatments can be extremely effective, some of the patients I could not help were getting pregnant with these other modalities. That made me question what else was out there, and reach out to some of those practitioners.

My discoveries inspired a new sense of wonderment and yearning in me to learn what else I could offer my patients; other than the traditional therapies I was taught in medical school. I had also seen so many miracles happen; so many patients become pregnant who were told they never could. This included those who had no sperm, whose tubes were blocked, who had severe scarring and disease surrounding their ovaries, or who simply "gave up." I learned to never say never again, based on my own personal experience, and the experiences of those for whom I was caring. These miracles made me wonder—is there more?

I had the pleasure of meeting many wonderful naturopaths who taught me the value of our lifestyle choices and that we are in fact what we eat. Our bodies can only use the building blocks we give them to make us healthy. I also believe in supporting the practice, education and research of a healing and prevention-based approach to health and well-being. As we are learning more and more today, food is medicine. Dr. Wylde's chapter focuses on how to improve your fertility from a naturopathic perspective. She is a naturopathic doctor working in Vaughan, Ontario, Canada. I approached her to be a part of this book because she has looked after and worked with my patients in an intelligent, caring and compassionate manner over the past several years. She has demonstrated unparalleled clinical acumen and has worked closely with me in caring for our mutual patients. She is a wonderful asset to my work, with a comprehensive understanding of herbal remedies that I don't have, and which complements my treatment strategy.

At my first clinic, I introduced a group of acupuncturists and traditional Chinese medicine doctors to my medical peers, and we integrated them into the clinic as part of our team. Dr. Tanaka's chapter will explain how acupuncture and East Asian medicine can be of value in reproductive health. I have had the pleasure of knowing Dr. Tanaka since 2007, when I first started working as a gynecologic reproductive endocrinologist and infertility specialist in downtown Toronto. We have a deep mutual respect and we have cared for many of our patients together. Dr. Tanaka is a renowned acupuncturist and Asian medicine doctor whom I admire greatly and whose expertise with these techniques complements my Western medical approach.

After I moved to my second clinic, I encountered a health challenge that I just could not fathom, or make any sense of using the traditional medical model. My nurse at the time introduced me to a trainer of neurolinguistic programming (NLP). I also met with a chiropractor who was practicing German New Medicine, while I continued to seek the help of Western medical doctors. With all of these modalities combined, I was able to help my body heal itself.

With this fantastic development in my own health, I went on to pursue further learning and became a certified NLP trainer, a certified NLP master coach, and a school of hypnosis and master practitioner of Time Line Therapy™. At my own clinic, I incorporated the services of mind-body coaches into our patients' care, if that was their wish. You can read more about the mind-body connection, and its power in Glenda Johnson's chapter on mind-body awareness. I have known Glenda since I took my hypnosis training in 2011. She has been not only a colleague who has helped my patients, but she has also been coaching me throughout my personal and professional efforts. I have learned more about myself and others from her than from anyone else so far. Her advanced mind-body techniques have helped my patients identify underlying limiting beliefs and trapped energies, that when released allowed them to have a clearer vision of what they needed to achieve their goals.

As anyone who has gone through this journey knows, it can be extremely emotionally draining and the support of one another, your friends and family, and in some situations, a fertility counselor, can make a world of difference when things seem hopeless. In her chapter, Reina Zatylny outlines how a counselor's support and expertise can help you through the ups and downs of the fertility roller coaster, and help you find hope in the depths of despair. Reina is a counselor with whom I have worked for almost 10 years. She has been instrumental in helping my patients during times of emotional turmoil and heartache using EMDR (eye movement desensitization and reprocessing techniques) in order to deal with past issues and current phobias (such as fear of needles), and has always been there when any of them needed her. Her compassion and passion for what she does is immeasurable.

I have been working with fertility patients for over 15 years and have been lucky enough to have helped thousands of them achieve their dreams of a family, while also supporting those that did not always get what they wanted. In going through fertility treatments myself, I learned all too well, what the medical treatments were all about, everything from the least to the most invasive. I am honored to have the opportunity to share a little bit about them with you in my chapter.

The medical treatment of fertility has developed to levels where we can achieve incredible results, although they do come with complications in a small percentage of cases. The successes are incredibly rewarding, and the highs are super high, however, the lows are truly devastating, to patients and doctors alike. New technologies and new treatments continue to be developed, which propel us towards continually improving outcomes. In my chapter, I summarize the current options for medical treatment, though it is by no means an exhaustive review. It is meant to give you an overview of your options, which you can then discuss with your physician, who can provide you further tailored and personalized care based on your particular situation.

The thought of having a partner with no sperm, or being a single woman, or a lesbian couple looking at your options may seem a bit overwhelming at first. However, the easy to understand and practical approach outlined by Haimant Bissessar in his chapter, will make you feel much more at ease as you navigate your path to finding your ideal donor sperm. Each clinic and sperm bank will also have a health professional who can guide you through the process easily and effortlessly. Haimant has been an avid advocate of sperm donation since the day I met him. He has worked in the field of assisted reproductive technologies for thirty years, and is extremely supportive of patients who may be considering or needing donor sperm. He stands out to me because he is always looking for new ways to incorporate more and more options for our mutual patients and is always happy to help.

A fertility challenge is certainly not something anyone plans for, prepares for, or expects. This is especially true when you realize that your own pool of eggs may have diminished in number and/or quality, and that you may need to consider using another woman's eggs to have a baby. Or, you may realize that your uterus may not be able to carry a pregnancy. It rocks your foundation and makes you question your womanhood. Coming to terms with these biological and psychological concepts is the first hurdle, however, once you do, you are able to realize that there are options that are extremely effective. These are outlined by David Sher in his chapter.

The availability of frozen eggs, and agencies that coordinate these services, has truly revolutionized this type of fertility care. The first time I met David, we had an instant connection in our fervent effort to help our patients. His beaming smile and boundless heart were evident immediately. He has gone above and beyond to help my patients who have needed an egg donor, and we have been working together immensely well. His depth of knowledge regarding egg donation is beyond my scope and he continues to stay current and ahead of newly developing science in this area that allows patients to get the best possible chance of success.

Adoption may be the choice you make for building your family. Sofie Stergianis demystifies this process and walks you through it with clarity and sensitivity. As with any of the options discussed, this is a choice that not everyone will feel comfortable with, however, if you do, it is an incredible gift for both you and the child you adopt. Sofie is a private adoption professional who I met through a recommendation from one of my patients. Though we have not met in person, the moment we connected on the phone, I knew she was the perfect choice for this chapter and book. She is a fervent advocate of adoption and her attention to detail was evident throughout this project.

It has been my dream and hope to complete this book for many years now, because I have seen my patients work through the ups and downs of the fertility roller coaster. Having been on it myself, I respect and honor each and every one's personal and unique experience. No two of us are the same, and I strive to help you in a way that serves your needs wherever you are on your journey.

My aim was to put together a resource for those of you who are experiencing challenges in building a family. You may choose one path, or you may combine several. Your options are many.

Please enjoy reading about all the tools you can access to help you succeed, and come join us on your journey!

Chapter 1: Naturopathic Medicine

A Couple's Struggle—For a Reason You Won't Believe;

by David and Sandra MacDonald

Like most couples with infertility, my wife and I have a story to share about our struggle to conceive. In our case, it took six years.

My name is David. My wife Sandra and I have been married for nine-and-a-half years and live in Toronto, Canada, where we are both sales professionals. We take a lot of pride in what we eat and we exercise regularly. In October 2009, after living and working abroad in Singapore and New York City for a combined four-and-a-half years, we returned to Toronto to settle down and start a family. Sandra was thirty-two and I was thirty-six, and we were feeling pressure from our families to have our first baby.

We had a lot on our minds when we first started trying because we were overthinking everything—the right position, time of the month, even the type of moon. It became stressful and confusing. In the summer of 2010, we began to learn about health and wellness along with alternative medicines, and we were fascinated by the stories we read about people being healed without pharmaceutical drugs, hospitals, and doctors. That's when we decided to dig deeper into treatments that could assist our bodies with conception.

Sandra eventually sourced an acupuncturist in downtown Toronto who we'll refer to as "Jane" for her privacy. Jane began by prescribing a wide range of herbal teas and pills for us to take while we received acupuncture treatment on a weekly basis for the next eleven months. The frequent changes in our plans got tiring. I remember by the end how angry and emotionally drained we felt after all the time, money, and trust we put into someone who didn't have the expertise we needed. I felt a lot of pain for Sandra as she started to blame herself for not being able to provide us with a baby. It was a terrible feeling of emptiness and sadness which almost dragged both of us into depression.

In the spring of 2011, Sandra suggested that we be tested for infertility and learn about the scientific methods available to us. Our first appointment was at a fertility clinic in downtown Toronto that had a glowing reputation for helping couples with infertility. They first tested our blood and my sperm for deficiencies and abnormalities. When the results came in, the fertility doctor informed us that everything was good; however, some of my sperm were considered poor quality, which they said was normal as most men don't have perfect sperm. We were reminded that we only needed one good sperm to make its way to Sandra's eggs.

Our counselor advised us of the options we had which included intrauterine insemination (IUI) and in vitro fertilization (IVF). It was explained that IUI is a form of assisted conception, which meant our doctor would place washed, prepared sperm from me into Sandra's uterus at her time of ovulation. This procedure required Sandra to take fertility drugs to increase her chances of conceiving. The counselor said that the success rate for this procedure at Sandra's age of thirty-four was about 10 percent per attempt. Next to consider was IVF. We were amazed when they explained that the IVF involved removing Sandra's eggs from her ovaries and mixing them with my sperm in a laboratory where conception took place in a sterile dish. The success rate for this procedure was much higher with IVF.

We talked about and debated IUI versus IVF. We could use IUI, which cost a few hundred dollars but had lower success rates, or we could spend upwards of $15,000 for IVF with the greater chance of ending our struggles and fulfilling our dream of having our first baby. Both procedures involved taking fertility drugs, which concerned us; we weren't clear if it was a necessity and we didn't know the possible long-term effects it could have on Sandra's health. After talking things over for a couple of weeks, we decided to try the IUI without the assistance of medications. A few weeks later we learned that Sandra was not pregnant. We strongly resisted the clinic's recommendations for us to have a drug assisted IUI or IVF and didn't want another opinion. We were back to square one and feeling frustrated.

I decided to take Sandra on a vacation to take our minds off things and lift our spirits, given the emotional toll this was taking on us. In September 2012, we conceived for the first time only to lose the baby a few weeks later. One evening Sandra and I cried for hours, resigning ourselves to the fact that we needed help on many levels as our bodies and minds were exhausted from the stress of failing ourselves. Later that month, Sandra decided to find us a reputable infertility expert that specialized in natural healing and wellness practices. Eventually, she discovered a renowned naturopathic doctor recognized for her expertise in women's health, acupuncture, pregnancy, and fertility.

Initially Sandra met with the doctor herself to determine if she liked her and to assess if her approach to fertility was in line with our desire to be helped naturally. The doctor was very empathetic to the fact that Sandra had just miscarried after three years of trying and gave Sandra renewed hope that she would get pregnant again. The doctor started by prescribing some supplements to support Sandra's egg quality and ran a bunch of blood tests. Sandra returned to this doctor in early January 2013, five-and-a-half weeks pregnant. Unfortunately, she miscarried one week later. A few weeks after that, we found out for the first time that Sandra had an excellent ovarian reserve (lots of eggs).

The doctor decided to run more tests to rule out any autoimmune or hormone problems. Sandra's thyroid was healthy, and there was no underlying autoimmune problem, but her didehydroepiandrosterone (DHEA) and progesterone were low. The doctor was away on maternity leave from April 2013 to January 2014, so we decided to try another fertility clinic and attempted two more IUI's, both with no success. Sandra had another miscarriage in December 2013. We returned to our naturopathic doctor in January 2014 to receive the complementary support that would prepare us for an IVF procedure. After my consultation and testing, we learned that my sperm count was good, although my sperm motility (movement) and morphology (shapes) were compromised. I also had elevated sperm antibodies. The doctor zeroed in on a childhood surgery I had had for varicose veins in my leg and suggested an ultrasound to rule out the possibility of a varicocele.

Sandra and I were relieved to receive this advice because now we could develop a plan to address what was impeding our ability to conceive. Our doctor started giving us acupuncture on a weekly basis to treat Sandra for her spleen qi deficiency and me for my liver blood stasis (a traditional Chinese medicine diagnosis). She also had us follow a strict diet that excluded all flours, sugars, and alcohol to help us drop some weight and improve the circulation to our reproductive organs. In addition, we were put on supplement programs to protect our bodies against oxidative stress. Quickly, this became a regimented lifestyle that required a lot of discipline. Our bodies were raging with disapproval when we first cut sugar and flour out of our diet, and it was approximately three weeks before we stopped craving them and were able to normalize our days. The acupuncture techniques our doctor used were unlike anything we experienced before as she focused a lot on reducing our stress in addition to addressing our individual traditional Chinese medicine diagnoses. It made us feel balanced and our bodies functioned in a more optimal way for the things we noticed such as better digestion, improved moods, and deeper sleep. We also had more mental clarity and improved energy levels. These changes were addictive and positive and gave us a deep desire to stay the course at any expense, as we felt we were in the right care and had the right mentor to guide us. Over time, the quality of my sperm started to improve and we knew that we were getting closer.

After consulting with our doctor, we went to the fertility clinic and requested an ultrasound on my testicles to rule out any problems before we proceed with an IVF. A few weeks later, in March 2014, the ultrasound was performed, after which a urologist diagnosed me with a severe varicocele. I learned that the varicocele was impeding the blood flow and oxygen to my testicles, which was believed to have a direct impact on the quality of my sperm. The doctor told me that a surgery could repair the varicocele but the recovery would take as long as twelve months. Sandra and I didn't want to wait twelve months and decided to go for it and do the IVF in June 2014 with medications. We felt we had a good chance to conceive given the improvements we had made in our health.

We agreed to have pre-implantation genetic screening (PGS) on our three blastocysts on day six, to ensure we used the strongest embryo for the transfer. After waiting a couple of weeks for the results, we were told that two of the blastocysts were deemed not compatible with life. The third was classified as zero result as there wasn't enough genetic material for the lab technician to say if it was healthy or not.

Sandra and I told the fertility clinic that we wanted to proceed with the transfer of the frozen blastocyst with undetermined health, in case it would further develop to a point where it would sustain itself within Sandra's uterus. In October 2014, Sandra had an early miscarriage following the frozen embryo transfer, which the fertility clinic attributed to Sandra's egg quality. We were frustrated, angry and sad, and we disagreed with their theory. Shortly after the news, I arranged to have my varicocele embolization and was fortunate enough to have it scheduled the next week at a Toronto hospital. I was awake for the procedure, which lasted an hour and was told by the doctors that they coiled off eight areas that were pooling blood into the testicle.

Over the next several months, our doctor focused on speeding up the healing of my varicocele given the biological time crunch we were facing. During that time, she referred us to a fertility doctor for consultation prior to us having another IVF. New tests revealed that Sandra's thyroid antibodies were now a problem, even though her thyroid hormones seemed healthy. This was frustrating as the endocrinologist informed us that it might have been a result of the medications from the first IVF. The fertility doctor told us that she would use a different protocol involving less medication to ensure we didn't over-stimulate Sandra's eggs, as she felt that this may have affected the quality of the earlier blastocysts. Our naturopath continued to treat us with acupuncture and switched our supplement protocol to include immune system support due to my anti-sperm antibodies and Sandra's thyroid antibodies. She also recommended that we continue taking our antioxidants for our sperm and egg quality.

One evening, while we were preparing for our second IVF, Sandra said, "What the heck, it's been seven months since your surgery, let's try naturally to see if we can nail it on our own." We were feeling really good about our treatments, along with the complementary strategies of our naturopath and our fertility doctor. On July 4, 2016, Sandra and I conceived naturally. Our fertility doctor was a great support from the beginning, monitoring Sandra through the first trimester to ensure she had adequate progesterone and thyroid levels, and performing periodic ultrasounds. We will always be grateful for her heartfelt dedication to go above and beyond to help us get through the first three months when she didn't have to.

As always, our naturopathic doctor was right there for Sandra, providing acupuncture treatments for improving blood flow to the uterus, reducing her stress levels, and advising her on so many things including nutrition and exercise. A few months after I wrote this passage, Sandra and I were blessed with the opportunity to be parents when our beautiful baby girl Alyssa Charlotte MacDonald was born at 10:07 a.m. March 22, 2016.

A special heartfelt thank you to our naturopathic doctor who was so strong for us, never allowing us to give in, keeping us focused, and giving us so much of her own energy throughout our conversations and treatments. Our baby girl will also want to thank you, and our fertility doctor, for all you have done!

How Naturopathic Medicine Can Help You Get Pregnant and Stay Pregnant;

by Dr. Tanya Wylde, ND, R.Ac

I am excited and honored to have been asked to write this chapter on how naturopathic medicine can help you through your fertility journey and achieve a healthy pregnancy. Many fertility clinics have incorporated integrative strategies of treatment by combining conventional assisted reproductive technologies (ART) with complementary approaches, such as naturopathic medicine and acupuncture, as the research literature continues to validate their efficacy in improving healthy pregnancy outcomes.[1]

This chapter will give you some of the most effective, evidence-informed lifestyle recommendations and natural medicine treatment approaches to improving fertility and ultimately achieving a healthy pregnancy, whether you are attempting to conceive naturally or with ART. In the last ten years, I have helped so many patients get pregnant with customized treatment programs and accurate diagnoses of their underlying obstacles to optimum fertility. Research suggests that eating healthy[2], supplementing appropriately[3], exercising regularly[4], and reducing stress levels[5] can improve your chances of achieving a healthy pregnancy. I will also reveal how naturopathic medicine can help with in vitro fertilization (IVF).

Taking a thorough history is crucial for me to ensure that you have been properly diagnosed and that I can optimize your fertility support. My goal is to help both you and your partner get into the best possible state of health by addressing any issues that might be contributing to your subfertility. As a naturopathic doctor (ND) and acupuncturist, I will assist you and your partner in achieving an ideal weight, optimal nutrient status, reduced stress levels, improved circulation to your reproductive system, and healthier sperm and egg quality. By improving these factors, you will have a better chance of attaining a healthy pregnancy outcome. Individualizing nutrition, supplement plans, exercise regimens and acupuncture protocols makes it possible for me to appropriately address all of your health conditions.

It can be difficult to know who to trust or turn to during your fertility journey. Incorporating an ND into your team of health care providers may reduce your chances of requiring multiple attempts at ART before achieving your goal of a healthy, successful pregnancy. Furthermore, NDs will support your physical and mental health throughout the process.

Weight

One of the most important factors contributing to healthy eggs and sperm is maintaining a healthy weight and fat percentage[6]. I always calculate you and your partner's body mass index (BMI) using standardized charts, and estimate fat percentages using a bio-impedance analysis machine. Carrying a BMI outside of the healthy range of 20 to 25 kg/ m^2 can adversely affect ovulation, as well as egg quality and sperm quality[7]. A BMI above 25 is considered overweight and above 30, obese. As toxins tend to be fat-soluble, those with higher body fat percentages will have higher toxic loads. Toxins in the form of endocrine disrupting chemicals (EDCs), such as Bisphenol-A and pesticides, are especially problematic as they may contribute to ovulation problems due to their undesired hormonal impact[8]. Carrying excess fat promotes the release of hormones, such as leptin and insulin, in addition to inflammatory cytokines[9]. This increases inflammation and oxidative stress, which affects egg and sperm quality much like smoking does[10]. Oxidative stress is the burden placed on you by your body's constant production of free radicals and by environmental stresses such as radiation, toxins, and tobacco smoke. Antioxidants neutralize the harmful activity of oxidants (free radicals). Good sperm and egg quality depends on a balance between oxidative stress and antioxidant defenses. Being overweight can also promote the growth of uterine fibroids and endometrial lesions, and can cause ovulation disruption in women with ovulation disorders. Being too thin or carrying an unhealthy low-fat percentage can also prevent or disrupt ovulation, as well as detrimentally affect your egg quality.[11]

In men, excess body fat and toxins may contribute to hormonal disturbances, increased scrotal temperatures, and adversely affect sperm quality and quantity. It doesn't mean that every overweight woman or man will have difficulty getting pregnant, or that weight loss will be your cure, but weight really can impact your fertility.[12]

Research suggests that pregnancy rates are lower in obese women undergoing in vitro fertilization (IVF) compared with women of healthy, normal weight[13].

Some of the proposed reasons for less successful IVF in overweight women include increased risk of treatment cancellation, limited ability to visualize the ovaries during ultrasound monitoring, more challenging egg retrieval, inferior egg quality, and impaired absorption of medication due to increased fat stores. Being overweight and pregnant is also associated with higher risks of miscarrying, hypertension, gestational diabetes, pre-eclampsia, severe low back pain, and labor complications.

Nutrition

The best diet for fertility is a non-processed one, emphasizing low glycemic index (GI) foods[14]. Consuming low GI foods helps you maintain healthier blood sugars. High GI foods have more added sugars and are more processed so they are less fertility-friendly and should be minimized. For example, whole fruits and vegetables should be emphasized over juices or dried options, and whole grains, such as brown rice or whole wheat, should be emphasized over white rice and white flour products. Similarly, unprocessed meats or fish such as roast beef or fish fillets are preferred over beef jerky and deep-fried and battered fish. You should also limit or avoid sweets and desserts.

A recent study (published in the American Journal of Clinical Nutrition) investigated the effects of a low calorie, low GI diet on unhealthy hormone concentrations that affect fertility and pregnancy rates in overweight and obese sub-fertile women undergoing IVF[15]. There were greater reductions in BMI, percentage body fat, waist-hip ratio, and the hormone leptin in the low GI diet group than in the control group. The low GI diet group experienced 85 percent more oocytes (mature eggs) retrieved, as well as more spontaneous pregnancies during follow-up. Although a higher BMI is implicated in reduced fertility, poor quality embryos have also been seen among thin and healthy women who eat a high carbohydrate, higher GI, lower protein diet. Evidence suggests that eating a diet with 25 percent more protein and 40 percent less carbohydrate, improves egg quality and doubles pregnancy rates in IVF, even among women who are slim and have a healthy BMI.

Two other studies, published in the *Journal of Human Reproduction*, found that pesticides (known as endocrine disrupting chemicals or EDCs) on fruits and vegetables could have a detrimental effect on your reproductive organs, hormones, and pathways[16]. In men, higher levels of EDCs were linked with poorer semen quality. Women with higher levels of EDCs in their follicular fluid had fewer follicles properly mature to eggs and fewer mature embryos at the end of the IVF process. This is why I want you to eat organic, pesticide-free foods and avoid chemical products on your body and in your home.

You can make the transition to organic foods by avoiding the Environmental Working Group's (EWG) "dirty dozen," which is a list of the top twelve foods with the most pesticide residues[17]. EWG is a non-profit American environmental organization specializing in toxic chemical research and advocacy. You can also choose healthier cosmetics and cleaning products (avoiding parabens, fragrances, and ingredients you don't recognize) by consulting their list of fertility-friendly products.[18]

You should limit or avoid alcohol and caffeine.[19] Consuming over 150 mg of caffeine per day increases your risk of miscarriage[20]. It can overstimulate the adrenals causing low-grade stress and suppress your appetite. If you miss the taste of coffee, try organic Swiss water decaffeinated coffee.

When you to go the grocery store, shop around the perimeter and select fresh produce, nuts, seeds, grass-fed meats, organic chicken, wild fish, and organic, healthy starches. Eat fruits low on the glycemic index and high in antioxidants such as berries, plums, peaches, nectarines, apricots, apples, and pears. Emphasize dark green leafy vegetables, which are full of fiber, minerals, and phytonutrients, including folic acid. Avoid flour products (pasta, breads, baked goods, crackers) and instead focus on healthier starches like brown rice, quinoa, root vegetables (such as sweet potatoes, carrots, beets, turnips, squash) and legumes (kidney beans, lentils, lima beans, chickpeas, etc.).

Dietary fat intake has also been studied for its effect on reproductive health. Trans-fats have been associated with ovulatory infertility and miscarriages, while saturated fats have been associated with lower sperm concentrations, lower egg and embryo quality, and inferior pregnancy outcome in IVF[21]. Foods high in saturated fats, such as French fries, chips, and red meats, can also increase inflammation and aggravate endometriosis. Choose organic eggs and dairy products and get tested for dairy sensitivity in cases of autoimmune subfertility. Choose extra lean beef and red meats that have been grass fed, or game meats like bison and elk that are leaner and healthier since they are typically fed a more natural diet. Eat healthy fats with meals, such as coconut and olive oils, avocados, nuts, and seeds.

Selecting healthier fish is also important. Fish makes a healthy protein option but choose fish that are higher in omega-3 fats and lower in mercury. Good choices include wild Alaskan salmon, canned salmon, Atlantic mackerel,

Pacific sardines, Atlantic or Pacific herring, rainbow trout, and snow crab legs. Avoid tuna, orange roughie, lobster, grouper, and snapper, since they have less essential fats or are higher in mercury. Excellent resources include the Environmental Defense Fund seafood selector and the EWG seafood calculator. When trying to conceive, I recommend up to three servings per week, plus an omega-3 fatty acid supplement, since increased omega-3 fatty acid intake has been shown in studies to improve embryo morphology and quality during the IVF cycle.[22]

Egg and Sperm Quality and Healthy Hormone Balance

One of the most significant factors affecting your fertility is your egg quality. Today, more women are choosing to have children later in life, but many women mistakenly believe that as long as they are healthy, they can delay childbirth without consequence. After the age of thirty-five there is a general decline in a woman's egg quality, with the biggest drop-off between the ages of thirty-eight and forty-two[23]. As you age, so do your eggs. If you try to conceive after the age of thirty-five, it may take longer and you are more likely to need help.

Men, however, create a new set of fully matured sperm every three months. This doesn't mean that their sperm will be perfect, as sperm are also susceptible to age-related oxidative stress and influenced by diet, medications, environment, lifestyle, and other factors[24]. I insist on semen analysis of male partners in order to identify any unhealthy sperm parameters, such as low sperm counts, poor motility and morphology, or a high degree of DNA fragmentation. You can improve both sperm and egg quality, but it takes time. Follicles go through a 90-day maturation process in the ovaries and sperm maturation can take between 70 and 90 days in the testicles. So over a three-month span we can work towards improving both your egg and his sperm quality, with improved circulation, nutrition, hormone balance, and antioxidant status regardless of your subfertility diagnosis.

Egg quality and hormone production are closely linked. To produce the optimum amount of hormones you need quality eggs. If the optimum amounts of hormones are produced, the likelihood of conceiving and sustaining a healthy pregnancy is higher on that given cycle. This also positively affects the quality of the remaining follicles that will grow and mature into eggs in future cycles.

Irregular menstrual cycles are a sign of a hormonal imbalance, which can compromise fertility. Research has shown that women with high menstrual cycle variability (early or late ovulation) have a reduced probability of pregnancy (51 percent lower per cycle) compared with women with minimal variability.[25]

I will likely test your blood for anti-Müllerian hormone (AMH), prolactin, dehydroepiandrosterone (DHEA) free testosterone, fasting cortisol, fasting insulin, and thyroid hormone levels. Testing your AMH provides information concerning your ovarian reserve—how many eggs you have left. A low AMH for your age could indicate premature ovarian insufficiency (POI). A high AMH for your age likely indicates polycystic ovarian syndrome (PCOS). A healthy AMH level for your age does not necessarily mean that your follicles are perfect quality. I may also measure certain hormones at specific times of the menstrual cycle, including follicle-stimulating hormone (FSH), estradiol, and progesterone.

Optimal thyroid hormone balance is also related to a healthy menstrual cycle and improved fertility[26]. I usually assess several of your thyroid hormones, including thyroid-stimulating hormone (TSH), free T3, and free T4. If I suspect that your thyroid is being attacked by your immune system, I will test your levels of thyroid antibodies, specifically anti-thyroperoxidase and anti-thyroglobulin. An acceptable TSH level for the general population is less than 5.0, but a value of less than 2.5 is the new standard for optimal fertility. Ideally, your free T3 and free T4 levels should be in the upper two-thirds of the healthy range. Make sure that your prenatal vitamin supplement has at least 150 mcg of iodine to support your thyroid[27]. Pregnant women need more iodine because of increased thyroid hormone production and fetal iodine requirements. Iodine deficiency during pregnancy can result in increased likelihood of pregnancy loss and severe health problems with the baby, including intellectual impairment[28]. Too much iodine, however, can actually suppress thyroid function.[29]

One method of addressing age-related subfertility is supplementation with antioxidants. Co-enzyme Q10 (CoQ10) is my favorite antioxidant that can help both you and your partner's reproductive health, regardless of your age and your fertility diagnosis[30]. CoQ10 improves the function of the energy-producing mitochondria found within eggs and sperm, which is key to optimizing quality. Melatonin, another potent antioxidant, has been found to improve egg and embryo quality in women undergoing IVF.

I may also recommend phytoestrogenic herbs such as black cohosh and red clover (which act like a low dose of estrogen), and phytoprogestogenic herbs such as wild yam and chasteberry (which act like a low dose of progesterone), especially if your menstrual cycles are becoming shorter or irregular. These herbs are especially helpful when your menstrual cycle is irregular since they can improve hormone levels and egg quality, thus improving menstrual regularity. If your blood DHEAs levels are low, I might recommend supplementing with this potent antioxidant because it has been shown to reduce chromosome problems in the embryo resulting in lower miscarriage rates.[31]

For men with poor sperm parameters, I recommend various antioxidants, such as CoQ10, L-carnitine, acetyl-L-carnitine, N-acetylcysteine (NAC), vitamin E, vitamin C, beta-carotene, zinc, omega-3, and folic acid[32]. I also address underlying causes of male factor infertility, including smoking, obesity, poor diet, stress, and/or poor circulation from a varicocele (varicose vein in the testicles).

Your egg quality may be affected by age, or by certain underlying conditions such as PCOS. Various supplements including NAC, myo-inositol and berberine have been shown in double-blind, placebo-controlled studies to improve egg quality, menstrual cycle regularity, and clinical pregnancy rates in women with PCOS[33]. These supplements can also reduce levels of excess circulating androgens (male hormones) and improve insulin resistance, which has been identified as a potential underlying cause of PCOS, even in thin women with the condition.

Circulation, Healthy Sperm and Endometrial Lining

Almost half of all men with subfertility will have an associated varicocele that is reducing circulation to the testicles[34]. A man needs healthy circulation to his testicles to produce optimal sperm parameters: sperm counts, motility, normal sperm morphology, and reduced DNA fragmentation (levels of oxidative stress on the sperm). A varicocele can be identified by physical examination and ultrasound. There is conflicting evidence that surgical repair to a varicocele will improve pregnancy outcome, but it significantly improves abnormal sperm parameters[35]. I might encourage surgery if your partner has a moderate to severe varicocele causing increased DNA fragmentation levels, even if you are planning IVF with intracytoplasmic sperm injection (ICSI)[36]. I also recommend acupuncture, improved nutrition, achieving a healthy weight, and antioxidants to speed up the healing process while continuing to work on improving sperm parameters[37]. It can take from six to twelve months post-surgery to see improvement.

You also need good blood flow to your uterus and ovaries for optimal endometrial lining thickness, embryo implantation, and improved egg quality. I often recommend supplements such as L-arginine to improve your circulation. If you are overweight, losing weight will help to improve circulation.

Physical exercise and acupuncture improve blood flow to your ovaries, your uterus, and your partner's testicles[38]. It is important not to over-exercise because this increases oxidative stress and adversely affects egg and sperm quality. I discourage couples from running marathons or long-distance triathlons for this reason. The right exercise program for you depends on your current BMI, fitness, fat percentage, and stress levels. A brisk walk for 30 to 60 minutes daily and yoga twice per week is a good start.

Autoimmune Conditions and Unexplained Infertility

Many of the changes we make to your lifestyle will help even if you have been diagnosed with "unexplained infertility," which may indicate that you have an undiagnosed autoimmune condition. For example, your thyroid stimulating hormone (TSH) levels may be optimal for fertility, but your antibodies to your thyroid may be positive. When you are pregnant, your immune system is weaker and having positive thyroid antibodies puts you at increased risk of early miscarriage (between four and eight weeks) and/or developmental problems with your baby. Researchers have found that women who suffer from high levels of thyroid antibodies may have reduced egg quality or early premature ovulation insufficiency (POI) because the thyroid antibodies may attack the eggs within your ovaries, in addition to the thyroid. If your thyroid antibodies are high, taking thyroid hormone medication while pregnant can help reduce your chances of miscarriage. I would also consider reducing your thyroid antibodies with selenomethionine, as indicated in the research literature[39].

Vitamin D3 supplementation may be necessary, as low levels of vitamin D3 have been found to be more prevalent in women with Hashimoto's (autoimmune) thyroiditis[40]. Higher vitamin D3 levels found in the follicular fluid of women undergoing IVF have resulted in higher clinical pregnancy rates compared with women with lower levels.[41]

If you are younger than thirty-five and are experiencing shorter menstrual cycles and earlier ovulation, it is important for me to identify whether you have an autoimmune condition that could be affecting your egg quality, ovarian reserve, or implantation, especially if you have had recurring pregnancy losses. Pre-implantation genetic screening (PGS) of your embryos created by IVF can be extremely useful in this situation. Recurring pregnancy losses with healthy embryos (as determined by PGS) indicates that you may have an autoimmune condition preventing their successful implantation.

Addressing your immune system imbalances with naturopathic medicine would include improving nutrition and circulation, specific antioxidants, digestion support, and stress management. Gastrointestinal health is critical because a large portion of your immune system is found within your gut. You can improve its health by removing pro-inflammatory foods from your diet and curing any infections (such as H. pylori and Candida), restoring healthy bacteria levels, and regenerating damaged portions of your intestinal lining due to ulcers, celiac disease, leaky-gut, etc[42]. I typically recommend fifty billion CFU of probiotics daily to modulate your immune system. Frequently rotating brands and types of probiotics will give you a variety of all species, subspecies and strains for optimal immune function. Depending on your condition, my individualized immune support plan for you could contain any of the following supplements: vitamin D, selenium, omega-3 fish oils, NAC, maritime pine bark, EGCG (an extract of green tea) and resveratrol (a potent antioxidant found in grapes). Addressing low DHEAs and progesterone levels can also help.

All women should take a prenatal multivitamin with the methyltetrahydrofolate (5-MTHF) form of folic acid in case they have an inherited genetic mutation that does not allow their bodies to absorb folic acid properly. Folic acid metabolism disorders can contribute to increased clotting, disruptions in the maturation process of your follicles (eggs), and difficulties with implanting and maintaining a healthy pregnancy[43]. Your fertility doctor can test you for this genetic mutation and other autoimmune conditions.

Unexplained infertility accompanied by severely painful periods requiring large doses of ibuprofen (Advil, Motrin) each month may lead me to suspect that you have endometriosis. Endometriosis is associated with lesions (endometrial glands) outside the uterus, often in the ovaries, that grow when your estrogen levels rise. Endometriomas create a lot of inflammation, reduce egg quality, and make implantation difficult[44]. Avoiding saturated fats, eating gluten-free, and taking omega-3 fats high in eicosapentaenoic acid (EPA) can reduce the inflammation associated with endometriosis[45]. Preliminary research has found that the antioxidant supplements N-acetylcysteine (NAC), EGCG, resveratrol, and pine bark can modulate the growth of endometriomas[46]. Increasing your antioxidant levels may shrink the lesions and improve your symptoms.

Stress

Every month that you do not get pregnant may bring up a multitude of emotions, including sadness, depression, and even jealousy. This can be extremely stressful, as can the daily cycle monitoring and fertility clinic visits if you are going through ART. You may feel disconnected from your family and friends because they are not as emotionally invested. A good social support network will help you get through this, as it is the number one predictor of good health. Keep your supportive friends close and work with health care experts such as naturopathic doctors, acupuncturists, and psychologists who specialize in fertility to help you emotionally.

It is imperative that you manage your stress hormones such as cortisol, which can contribute to oxidative stress levels and directly affect egg and sperm quality. Oxidative stress also increases your chances of miscarriage. In addition to weight gain and immune suppression, high cortisol from the adrenal glands (stress glands) sends messages to the brain to stop the healthy flow of fertility hormones, which can even suppress your ability to ovulate. Nature has wired us to be less fertile during famine and stressful situations for our protection.

We cannot always control the events that contribute to stress in our lives. However, we can change how we perceive and react to them. If you have optimal energy and are taking good care of yourself, your perception of stressful events improves. Start by working on improving your energy.

Regular exercise is an excellent stress reliever and can make you feel strong and energetic. In addition to cardiovascular exercise and weights, yoga is helpful because its focus on breathing and mindfulness is calming and nourishing. Eating healthy and every three hours to keep your blood sugar stable is also beneficial. Addressing nutrient deficiencies, such as low vitamin B12 and iron, and ensuring eight hours of sleep can improve your energy levels. Improving your energy and reducing your stress levels will improve your chances of pregnancy and reduce your chances of miscarriage.

Acupuncture combined with guided visual relaxation exercises are extremely effective at helping my patients feel calmer and more optimistic about achieving a healthy pregnancy. In studies, meditation and relaxation training have improved pregnancy rates by 30 percent in those undergoing fertility treatments.[47]

I also recommend that you continue to be intimate between ART cycles for two reasons. First, it may help you reconnect with your partner and reduce your stress, allowing for more enjoyable sex since the pressure of "trying" is off. Second, your body may still pick the right egg on a month off from fertility monitoring and ART cycles, no matter how many months or years that you have been trying. Never give up hope!

I hope that you have enjoyed reading this chapter on how naturopathic medicine can help you in your journey to getting pregnant and staying pregnant! I feel very fortunate to have had so many patients over the years trust me to make critical decisions around their health and pregnancy. Changing people's lives by helping them achieve their goal of having a baby is what fuels my determination to help the next couple that walks into my office. I am ready to help you and until we meet, remember to stay positive, surround yourself with the right people, and eat good, healthy foods. It's what your baby-to-be wants you to do!

---

[1] C.H. Zheng et al., "Effects of Acupuncture on Pregnancy Rates in Women Undergoing In Vitro Fertilization: A Systematic Review and Meta-Analysis," *Fertility and Sterility* 97, no. 3 (March 2012): 599-611, doi:10.1016/j.fertnstert.2011.12.007; R.S. Legro et al., "Randomized Controlled Trial of Preconception Interventions in Infertile Women with Polycystic Ovary Syndrome," *Journal of Clinical Endocrinology and Metabolism* 100, no. 11 (November 2015): 4048-58, doi:10.1210/jc.2015-2778.

[2] R. Sharma et al., "Lifestyle Factors and Reproductive Health: Taking Control of Your Fertility," *Reproductive Biology and Endocrinology* July 2013, doi:10.1186/1477-7827-11-66;2013;11:66; J.M. Twigt et al., "The Preconception Diet is Associated with the Chance of Ongoing Pregnancy in Women Undergoing IVF/ICSI Treatment," *Human Reproduction* 27, no. 8 (August 2012): 2526-31, doi:10.1093/humrep/des157; Gretchen Garbe Collins and Brooke V. Rossi, "The Impact of Lifestyle Modifications, Diet, and Vitamin Supplementation on Natural Fertility," *Fertility Research and Practice* 1, no. 11 (July 25, 2015), doi:10.1186/s40738-015-0003-4.

[3] K.J. Bühling and D. Grajecki, "The Effect of Micronutrient Supplements on Female Fertility," *Current Opinion in Obstetrics and Gynecology* 25, no. 3 (June 2013): 173-80, doi: 10.1097/GCO.0b013e3283609138; P. Gharagozloo, and R.J. Aitken, "The Role of Sperm Oxidative Stress in Male Infertility and the Significance of Oral

Antioxidant Therapy," Human Reproduction 26, no. 7 (July 2011): 1628-40, doi:10.1093/humrep/der132.
[4] Collins and Rossi, "The Impact of Lifestyle Modifications."
[5] C.D. Lynch et al., "Preconception Stress Increases the Risk of Infertility: Results from a Couple-Based Prospective Cohort Study—the LIFE Study," *Human Reproduction* 29, no. 5 (May 2014): 1067-75, doi:10.1093/humrep/deu032.
[6] M. Metwally, W.L. Ledger, and T.C. Li, "Reproductive Endocrinology and Clinical Aspects of Obesity in Women," *Annals of the New York Academy of Science* 1127 (April 2008): 140-6, doi:10.1196/annals.1434.000.
[7] Collins and Rossi, "The Impact of Lifestyle Modifications."
[8] E.M. Petro et al., "Endocrine-Disrupting Chemicals in Human Follicular Fluid Impair In Vitro Oocyte Developmental Competence," *Human Reproduction* 27, no. 4 (April 2012): 1025-33, doi:10.1093/humrep/der448; X. Huo et al., "Bisphenol-A and Female Infertility: A Possible Role of Gene-Environment Interactions," *International Journal of Environmental Research and Public Health* 12, no. 9 (September 2015): 11101-16, doi: 10.3390/ijerph120911101.
[9] G.F. Becker, E.P. Passos, and C.C. Moulin, "Short-Term Effects of a Hypocaloric Diet with Low Glycemic Index and Low Glycemic Load on Body Adiposity, Metabolic Variables, Ghrelin, Leptin, and Pregnancy Rate in Overweight and Obese Infertile Women: A Randomized Controlled Trial," *American Journal of Clinical Nutrition* 102, no. 6 (December 2015): 1365-72, doi:10.3945/ajcn.115.117200; P. Manna and S.K. Jain, "Obesity, Oxidative Stress, Adipose Tissue Dysfunction, and the Associated Health Risks: Causes and Therapeutic Strategies," *Metabolic Syndrome Related Disorders* 13, no. 10 (December 2015): 423-44, doi:10.1089/met.2015.0095.
[10] Y.H. Chiu et al., "Fruit and Vegetable Intake and Their Pesticide Residues in Relation to Semen Quality Among Men from a Fertility Clinic," *Human Reproduction* 2015 30, no. 6 (June 2015): 1342-51, doi:10.1093/humrep/dev064.
[11] N. Maconochie et al., "Risk Factors for First Trimester Miscarriage—Results from a UK-Population-Based Case-Control Study," *An International Journal of Obstetrics and Gynecology* 114, no. 2 (February 2007): 170-86.
[12] J.E. Chavarro et al., "Body Mass Index in Relation to Semen Quality, Sperm DNA Integrity, and Serum Reproductive Hormone Levels Among Men Attending an Infertility Clinic," *Fertility and Sterility* 93, no. 7 (May 2010): 2222-31, doi:10.1016/j.fertnstert.2009.01.100.
[13] S. Pandey et al., "The Impact of Female Obesity on the Outcome of Fertility Treatment," *Journal of Human Reproductive Sciences* 3, no. 2 (May-August 2010): 62-67, doi:10.4103/0974-1208.69332.
[14] Becker, Passos and Moulin, "Short-Term Effects of a Hypocaloric Diet."
[15] Becker, Passos and Moulin, "Short-Term Effects of a Hypocaloric Diet."
[16] Petro et al., "Endocrine-Disrupting Chemicals"; Chiu et al.,"Fruit and Vegetable Intake."
[17] Environmental Working Group, www.ewg.org/foodnews.summary.php.
[18] Environmental Working Group, www.ewg.org/skindeep/.
[19] G. Anifandis et al., "The Impact of Cigarette Smoking and Alcohol Consumption on Sperm Parameters and Sperm DNA Fragmentation (SDF) Measured by

Halosperm®," *Archives of Gynecology and Obstetrics* 290, no. 4 (October 2014): 777-82, doi: 10.1007/s00404-014-3281-x.

[20] J. Li et al., "A Meta-Analysis of Risk of Pregnancy Loss and Caffeine and Coffee Consumption During Pregnancy," *International Journal of Gynaecology and Obstetrics* 130, no. 2 (August 2015): 116-22, doi:10.1016/j.ijgo.2015.03.033.

[21] J.E. Chavarro et al., "Trans Fatty Acid Intake is Inversely Related to Total Sperm Count in Young Healthy Men," *Human Reproduction* 29, no. 3 (March 2014): 429-40, doi:10.1093/humrep/det464.

[22] F. Hammiche et al., "Increased Preconception Omega-3 Polyunsaturated Fatty Acid Intake Improves Embryo Morphology," *Fertility and Sterility* 95, no. 5 (April 2011): 1820-3, doi:10.1016/j.fertnstert.2010.11.021.

[23] K. Liu and Allison Case, "Advanced Reproductive Age and Fertility," *Journal of Obstetrics and Gynaecology Canada* 33, no. 11 (Nov 2011): 1165-75, http://sogc.org/wp-content/uploads/2013/01/gui269CPG1111E_000.pdf.

[24] P. Gharagozloo, and R.J. Aitken, "The Role of Sperm Oxidative Stress."

[25] C.M. Small et al.,"Menstrual Cycle Variability and the Likelihood of Achieving Pregnancy," *Reviews on Environmental Health* 25, no. 4 (Oct-Dec 2010): 369-78.

[26] A. Dave, L. Maru, and M. Tripathi, "Importance of Universal Screening for Thyroid Disorders in First Trimester of Pregnancy," *Indian Journal of Endocrinology and Metabolism* 18, no. 5 (September 2014): 735-8, doi:10.4103/2230-8210.139221.

[27] Bühling and Grajecki, "The Effect of Micronutrient Supplements."

[28] S.G. Obican et al., "Teratology Public Affairs Committee Position Paper: Iodine Deficiency in Pregnancy," *Birth Defects Research Part A: Clinical and Molecular Teratology* 94, no. 9 (September 2012): 677-82, doi:10.1002/bdra.23051.

[29] 29 A.M. Leung et al., "Potential Risks of Excess Iodine Ingestion and Exposure: Statement by the American Thyroid Association Public Health Committee," *Thyroid* 25, no. 2 (February 2015): 145-6, doi:10.1089/thy.2014.0331.

[30] G. Balercia et al., "Coenzyme Q10 Treatment in Infertile Men with Idiopathic Asthenozoospermia: A Placebo-Controlled, Double-Blind Randomized Trial," *Fertility and Sterility* 91, no. 5 (May 2009): 1785-92, doi:10.1016/j.

[31] N. Gleicher, A. Weghofer, and D.H. Barad, "Dehydroepiandrosterone (DHEA) Reduces Embryo Aneuploidy: Direct Evidence from Preimplantation Genetic Screening (PGS)," *Reproductive Biology and Endocrinology* 8 (November 2010): 140, doi 10.1186/1477-7827-8-140.

[32] E. Walczak-Jedrzejowska, J.K. Wolski, and J. Slowikowska-Hilczer,"The Role of Oxidative Stress and Antioxidants in Male Fertility," *Central European Journal of Urology* 66, no. 1 (April 2013): 60-7, doi:10.5173/ceju.2013.01.art19.

[33] Y. An et al., "The Use of Berberine for Women with Polycystic Ovary Syndrome Undergoing IVF Treatment," *Clinical Endocrinology (Oxford)* 80, no. 3 (March 2014): 425-31, doi:10.1111/cen.12294; D. Thakker et al., "N-Acetylcysteine for Polycystic Ovary Syndrome: A Systematic Review and Meta-Analysis of Randomized Controlled Clinical Trials," *Obstetrics and Gynecology International* (2015), doi:10.1155/2015/817849; V. Unfer et al., "Effects of Myo-Inositol in Women with PCOS: A Systematic Review of Randomized Controlled Trials," *Gynecology and Endocrinology* 28, no. 7 (July 2012): 509-15, doi:10.3109/09513590.2011.650660.

[34] Y.J. Wang et al., "Relationship Between Varicocele and Sperm DNA Damage and the Effect of Varicocele Repair: A Meta-Analysis," *Reproductive Biomedicine Online* 25, no. 3 (Sep 2012): 307-14, doi:10.1016/j.rbmo.2012.05.002.
[35] Ibid
[36] S.C. Esteves, F.V. Oliveira, and R.P. Bertolla, "Clinical Outcome of Intracytoplasmic Sperm Injection in Infertile Men with Treated and Untreated Clinical Varicocele," *Journal of Urology* 184, no. 4 (October 2010): 1442-6, doi:10.1016/j.juro.2010.06.004.
[37] J. Gual-Frau et al., "Oral Antioxidant Treatment Partly Improves Integrity of Human Sperm DNA in Infertile Grade I Varicocele Patients," *Human Fertility* 18, no. 3 (September 2015): 225-29, doi:10.3109/14647273.2015.
[38] E. Jedel et al., "Impact of Electro-Acupuncture and Physical Exercise on Hyperandrogenism and Oligo/Amenorrhea in Women with Polycystic Ovary Syndrome: A Randomized Controlled Trial*," American Journal of Physiology—Endocrinology and Metabolism* 300, no. 1 (January 2011): E37-45, doi:10.1152/ajpendo.
[39] L.H. Duntas, "Selenium and the Thyroid: A Close-Knit Connection*," The Journal of Clinical Endocrinology and Metabolism* 95, no. 12 (December 2010): 5180-8, doi:10.1210/jc.2010-0191.
[40] G. Tamer et al., "Relative Vitamin D Insufficiency in Hashimoto's Thyroiditis," *Thyroid* 21, no. 8 (August 2011): 891-6, doi:10.1089/thy.2009.0200.
[41] S. Ozkan et al., "Replete Vitamin D Stores Predict Reproductive Success Following In Vitro Fertilization," *Fertilility and Sterility* 94, no. 4 (September 2010): 1314-9, doi:10.1016/j.fertnstert.2009.05.019.
[42] E. Moretti et al., "Can Helicobacter Pylori Infection Influence Human Reproduction?" *World Journal of Gastroenterology* 20, no. 19 (May 2014): 5567-74, doi:10.3748/wjg.v20.i19.5567.
[43] K. Farahmand et al., "Thrombophilic Genes Alterations as Risk Factor for Recurrent Pregnancy Loss," *Journal of Maternal-Fetal and Neonatal Medicine* 29, no. 8 (April 2016): 1269-73, doi:10.3109/14767058.2015.1044431.
[44] C. Ngô et al., "Reactive Oxygen Species Controls Endometriosis Progression," *American Journal of Pathology* 175, no. 1 (July 2009): 225-34, doi:10.2353/ajpath.2009.080804.
[45] M. Marziali et al., "Gluten-Free Diet: A New Strategy for Management of Painful Endometriosis Related Symptoms?" *Minerva Chirugica* 67, no. 6 (December 2012): 499-504, http://www.minervamedica.it/en/journals/minervachirurgica/article.php?cod=R06Y2012N06A0499; M.M. Hopeman et al., "Serum Polyunsaturated Fatty Acids and Endometriosis," Reproductive Sciences 22, no. 9 (September 2015):1083-7. doi:10.1177/1933719114565030.
[46] A.G. Ricci et al., "Natural Therapies Assessment for the Treatment of Endometriosis," *Human Reproduction* 28, no. 1 (January 2013): 178-88, doi:10.1093/humrep/des369; H. Jr. Maia, C. Haddad, and J. Casoy, "Combining Oral Contraceptives with a Natural Nuclear Factor-Kappa B Inhibitor for the Treatment of Endometriosis-Related Pain," *International Journal of Women's Health* 6 (December

2013): 35-9, doi:10.2147/IJWH.S55210; C. Agostinis et al., "The Combination of N-Acetyl Cysteine, Alpha-lipoic acid, and Bromelain Shows High Anti-Inflammatory Properties in Novel In Vivo and In Vitro Models of Endometriosis," *Mediators of Inflammation* (2015), doi: 10.1155/2015/918089.

[47] A.D. Domar et al., "Impact of a Group Mind/Body Intervention on Pregnancy Rates in IVF Patients," *Fertility and Sterility* 95, no. 7 (June 2011): 2269-73, doi:10.1016/j.fertnstert.2011.03.046.

Chapter 2: Acupuncture and East Asian Medicine

Seven-Year Journey

My husband and I met when I was twenty-six and he was twenty-nine. After I finished my master's degree and my husband completed his engineering degree, he built a custom-made home with his own hands as a foundation to our marriage. We travelled. We had stable careers. We were healthy. We got married in 2005. I always wanted to have a family and all the pieces were in place, the timing was right. Six months later we officially started trying for a baby, but nothing could prepare me for the difficult seven-year journey ahead.

We tried—and tried—and tried. Month after month, nothing happened. Finally, after two years of trying, we were over the moon to receive a positive pregnancy test. We were so excited but the happiness was short lived when at about seven-and-a-half weeks I started to feel some minor cramping. I attributed it to normal stretching and growing. My family doctor sent me to the clinic to have ultrasounds. They found the pregnancy in my left Fallopian tube (an ectopic pregnancy) and that's when I was rushed to the hospital. I lost the baby but I was very lucky that my tube did not rupture. It was such a traumatic and shocking experience and three different nurses told me I was lucky to be alive. Losing that baby was absolutely heartbreaking.

I was advised to wait three months before trying to conceive again and the doctors told me that my chances of having a future successful pregnancy were very good. I took care of my health. Watched what I ate. Cut back on coffee and alcohol. But month after month I was becoming more discouraged. As the years went by and it didn't happen, we were devastated. After trying to start a family of our own for four years, a friend recommended acupuncture treatment.

At my very first acupuncture appointment in October 2009, I felt a new sense of hope. During that first consultation, I was asked a lot of questions. How was my sleeping? My menstrual cycle? Bowel movements? My diet? My acupuncturist looked at my tongue. Checked my pulse. Examined my eyes. I was also asked to track my diet for three days, with details of all food and beverages. Small diet changes were recommended such as cutting back on caffeine, no peaches or tofu that affected my thyroid, and a Chinese herbal formula to regulate my menstrual cycle, relax menstrual cramps, and ease indigestion. I also took prenatal vitamins and the omega-3 supplements EPA (eicosapentaenoic acid) and DHA (docosahexaenoic acid).

To my surprise, there were some other lifestyle changes that I was told would contribute to my improvement and help the proper circulation of blood and "qi," which, according to traditional Chinese medicine, is the life energy that circulates throughout the body. I was advised to minimize tight clothing and avoid overuse of pain medications. I was also advised to completely overhaul my inadequate diet by making more changes such as cutting out processed foods and eating more organic fruits and vegetables. The most difficult lifestyle change was making an effort to reduce the amount of computer time and time spent watching television after dinner, as I was told that the bright light from the screen affected quality of sleep. With our hectic jobs and day-to-day activities, keeping a regular pattern of sleep became a new priority in my life as I quickly discovered how sleep regulated my menstrual cycle.

After the first week of acupuncture treatment, I felt the positive effects immediately. I began to sleep soundly at night. I felt more energetic and relaxed during the day. Acupuncture reduced my stress and anxiety levels. It motivated me to go to the gym and strive to take better care of my health. My cravings for chocolate and other sugary sweets to combat that midday slump disappeared. The acupuncturist provided a quarterly newsletter with easy seasonal recipes I could try such as vegetarian Moroccan soup, sweet winter salad, and fall oatmeal cookies.

During the treatment, I was told that it was best to lightly close my eyes and think about something peaceful. Meditation music was played that always put me to sleep within five minutes. I always came out of my treatment session feeling rejuvenated. It felt like I was spending a day at the spa.

I am a person who feels queasy at the sight of regular needles. When I had my ears pierced, I fainted. The thought of acupuncture had me apprehensive but I had a number of friends who had success conceiving a child naturally with it. My acupuncturist quickly put my fears to rest. He used a Japanese acupuncture technique that was extremely gentle and painless. If anything, within five minutes I immediately felt washed over by a sense of relaxation and I fell asleep. For somebody who is always on-the-go, falling asleep so quickly is quite the accomplishment.

A form of heat treatment called "moxibustion" was also applied to stimulate specific acupuncture areas. This quickly became one of my favorite parts of the treatment, aside from the power nap. I found that the warm sensation applied to the acupuncture areas was actually quite soothing and more effective than having a massage. Along with the relaxing music to regulate my breathing, the soothing heat gave me the sensation of a peaceful escape, like basking in the warm sun on the beach. I began to look forward to my weekly treatments.

As part of my acupuncture, I was asked to track my basal body temperature on a chart every morning. It became a routine to check my temperature when first waking up in the morning and before getting out of bed. As my acupuncture treatments progressed, I quickly saw the positive results. Aside from my energy level being noticeably higher, I felt calmer and more peaceful. Within the first month, my cycle improved. It started to be like clockwork. Acupuncture helped to keep my cycle regular as I could see on my basal body temperature charts. Before treatment I used to experience very painful and nauseating periods that I had suffered from since high school. With weekly acupuncture sessions, I noticed my PMS symptoms disappeared. My periods became shorter and a regular twenty-eight days apart. I also noticed that my basal body temperature had a pattern. It was amazing to see and feel the changes.

After about six months of trying to conceive with acupuncture treatment, my acupuncturist strongly suggested that I have my blood work checked for my thyroid levels. That is when we discovered I have hypothyroidism. I was grateful that he encouraged me to test my thyroid level as that could be linked to my difficulty with fertility and the menstrual problems I had suffered from since high school. He also suggested that I see a fertility specialist. While I was on the waiting list to see the specialist, I continued to have weekly acupuncture and continued to see the positive results.

After only one cycle of being monitored at the fertility clinic we received the wonderful news that I was pregnant. After so many years of trying to conceive, we had never felt more ecstatic. It was like a dream. I remember my husband being so excited by the fantastic news given at the fertility clinic that he jumped out of his chair and hugged everybody he saw in the office. I stopped going for acupuncture. I had normal scans at eight weeks and twelve weeks and was told that everything was fine.

I felt a bit of pressure on my side but my obstetrician at the time said it was a growth pain. She booked an ultrasound for six weeks later. We were so excited about finding out the gender. Everything was going well until at about sixteen weeks, when I woke up at about one o'clock in the morning, and my world came crashing down. I was sleeping and woke up to a sudden gush of warm water. It was such a shock. My husband drove me to the hospital where I went into labor. I had my son that morning. It was the most difficult thing I have ever gone through and it is impossible to explain the magnitude of the loss.

Recovering from the dilation and curettage (D&C) to remove the pregnancy tissue and placenta from my uterus was painful both physically and emotionally, but instead of taking pain medication to help the cramping and ongoing bleeding, I went back to acupuncture. Not only did the acupuncture heal my body and quickly regulate my cycle, but it also eased the frustration, anger and depression from the loss. It helped me sleep soundly at night when I had insomnia, too. My family doctor was surprised by how quickly my body recovered from such a traumatic experience and said that we could try to conceive again after three months. I had a new sense of hope.

I continued to go to acupuncture weekly. After three months, I went back to the fertility clinic for cycle monitoring and the following cycle I received the wonderful news of positive results from blood work. That happiness was short lived. Sadly, a week later when I went for blood work, my hCG levels (pregnancy hormone) were dropping instead of increasing and I began bleeding. My family doctor told me it was twins.

My world turned upside down that same summer when my mother, my best friend, was diagnosed with stage four lung cancer. She never smoked a day in her life. She watched what she ate, did yoga and ran marathons. I thought she was the model of good health. By then I was too exhausted from the heartbreak of repeatedly losing hope of having a baby. I told the fertility clinic I was going to take a break from cycle monitoring to focus my energy on being with my mother who was in the hospital. One of the nurses at the fertility clinic advised me to have blood work the following cycle to see if my cycle was back on track and if my body was healing properly from the previous miscarriage. But by that point, I no longer had the energy. It was no longer a priority in my life.

Taking care of my mother and ensuring that she got the best treatment to fight cancer was my new battle. My cycle never came back. I didn't care. I gave up. A month went by. Then another. I did continue to have weekly acupuncture treatments between visits to the hospital. The acupuncture sessions helped me to deal with the stress and improved my quality of sleep when I had so many worries. It gave me the strength to tackle the most difficult time in my life and the clarity of mind to help my mother when she needed support the most.

I did notice that I missed my period but I just assumed my cycle was off because of the shock of my mother's sudden cancer diagnosis. After two months of not having a period, I saw my family doctor who confirmed through blood work that I was pregnant. This is a time when most people would be overjoyed by the news, but I was in disbelief. There were no symptoms. No cravings. No nausea. I was sleeping well. I can say that thanks to acupuncture, it felt relatively smooth.

This pregnancy was considered high-risk because of the previous losses. I was immediately referred to a high-risk pregnancy specialist where I had weekly appointments. From my very first ultrasound appointment, the specialist confirmed the baby was a boy. All that mattered to me was if the baby was healthy. Every week, I had the gift of seeing that tiny ultrasound. My weekly appointments were like a lifeline. Hearing that tiny heart beat was the best feeling in the world.

I continued acupuncture throughout the first trimester and part of the second trimester. Treatments helped prevent any morning sickness, back issues, cravings or other pregnancy complaints. My blood pressure was always normal and my glucose test was normal. Aside from it being a high-risk pregnancy, I felt great for most of the pregnancy and I attribute that to acupuncture. I had very few symptoms, which was amazing since my doctor put me on bed rest because I was diagnosed with an incompetent cervix. I had to stay off my feet and when I was home, I was lying down on the couch. No lifting. No climbing stairs. No standing to cook dinner or wash dishes. I had to take a leave of absence from work mid-second trimester to stay off my feet. At seventeen weeks I had a cerclage (a stitch to sew up my cervix) to prevent another preterm labor.

We were blessed with a very healthy and strong baby boy born on June 4, 2012. He was born full-term at thirty-six weeks, which was quite the accomplishment for a high-risk pregnancy and weak cervix. It is hard to believe that exactly one year earlier we were crying for our loss. After seven years of trying to have a baby and four miscarriages, we had given up on the dream of ever carrying a baby to term. We have so many people to thank who helped us along our journey. Special thank you to our talented doctors for helping us get to where we are today. Our little boy is a miracle and wouldn't have been possible without your knowledge and care.

We could never have predicted the overwhelming love and joy he has brought to our lives. He is now three years old, happy and thriving. He is also a talented musician thanks to the relaxation music that was regularly played during acupuncture while I was pregnant. Our little boy is truly our "Gift of God" and we treasure every day with him.

Acupuncture, East Asian Medicine, and Reproductive Health;

By Dr. Tim Tanaka, PhD., R.Ac, R.TCMP

For many decades, acupuncture has treated a variety of female reproductive issues in the East.[48] It has been widely used in the West, especially since the 1970s, for musculoskeletal pain conditions.[49] However, the application of acupuncture for other conditions, including reproductive health and fertility, has grown rapidly in recent years. Acupuncture use during in vitro fertilization (IVF) has sharply increased since 2002, when German researchers increased the success rate by nearly 50 percent in women undergoing IVF using acupuncture.[50]

Acupuncture can complement other conventional fertility therapies such as intrauterine insemination (IUI). You can also use it during the monitoring of your cycle, if you wish to conceive naturally without hormone drugs, or as a complementary treatment for underlying health conditions affecting your fertility such as endometriosis, uterine fibroids, ovarian cysts, polycystic ovary syndrome (PCOS), irregular menstruation, thin uterine lining, and hormonal imbalances.

In this chapter, I will discuss how acupuncture and traditional East Asian medicine can be beneficial for your reproductive health and increase your chance to conceive.

About Acupuncture

Acupuncture is a safe and effective natural therapy used to heal illness, prevent disease and improve well-being. Tiny, hair-thin needles are inserted into specific points in your body, where they are gently stimulated to trigger your body's natural healing response. Acupuncture is effective for controlling pain and can regulate your body's physiological functions to treat various internal dysfunctions and disorders.

Acupuncture was developed on the understanding that there are twelve main channels, or "regular meridians," running vertically, across, and throughout your body connecting the internal organs. It is a tenet of acupuncture that qi (somewhat equivalent to the western idea of vitality or life force) flows along these meridian lines.

The operating philosophy of traditional acupuncture is that disease is caused by interrupted energy flow at specific points on your body's surface. A needle is inserted at the affected point in order to stimulate qi flow and harmonize energy flow in your body. Points used may be at the site of the complaint or further away. Chinese medicine believes that good health requires a balance of forces in your body. Illnesses, pain and discomfort arise when the flow is blocked. The primary therapeutic intent of traditional acupuncture is to remove these blockages and restore the proper balance.

From the modern physiological perspective, one of the most well-known effects of acupuncture is the enhancement of blood flow. A number of human and animal studies have demonstrated the efficacy of acupuncture on circulatory systems in the skin, muscle, brain, and internal organs such as the ovaries and uterus.[51]

The potential effects of acupuncture on the female reproductive system

Acupuncture promotes the circulation of blood in the pelvic cavity and helps improve ovarian function. Studies have suggested that acupuncture treatment can be beneficial in promoting follicle production[52], enhancing uterine blood flow[53], and making the uterine lining more receptive to the implantation of an embryo.[54]

Acupuncture can be a useful and effective treatment if you are having difficulty conceiving without apparent cause (idiopathic infertility or so-called unexplained infertility). It can also be used to address a variety of health issues that create a potential barrier to you becoming pregnant, or as a complementary treatment for endometriosis, uterine fibroids, ovarian cysts, hypothyroidism, and various autoimmune conditions. Your response to acupuncture can vary depending on your health history and the severity of your condition.

How Acupuncture Works

Importance of blood flow to reproductive organs

Your circulatory system maintains efficient delivery of oxygen and nutrients to your organs and tissues, as well as the removal of metabolic waste. Disturbances of blood flow to your major arteries and vital organs can result in serious health consequences. Various organ dysfunctions, skin conditions, hormonal disorders, and symptoms such as being easily fatigued, lacking concentration, and becoming prone to injuries, are often associated with inadequate circulatory functions.

From the Chinese medicine perspective, proper flow of blood (and qi) is the most important factor for your body to function without pain or illness. Many female health concerns such as endometriosis, uterine fibroids, ovarian cysts, dysmenorrhea, and amenorrhea are often associated with Chinese medicine's diagnostic criterion of blood stasis (stagnation of old blood). Signs and symptoms of potential underlying circulation problems include cold hands and feet, varicose veins, painful menses, and clotted blood in your menstrual flow.

Increased blood flow to your ovaries and uterus enhances ovarian responsiveness and the development of adequate uterine lining for embryo implantation. Blood-thinning medications such as low-dose aspirin or heparin, sometimes prescribed by fertility specialists, are an example of a therapeutic attempt to increase blood flow in the uterine lining.[55] Some specialists have also been prescribing virginal sildenafil citrate (Viagra), in order to augment blood flow to female organs for women with thin uterine lining.[56] A series of laboratory experiments suggested that stimulating the body surface with acupuncture triggers a release of certain substances (such as calcitonin gene-related neuropeptide and substance P) that cause widening of blood vessels and increase of local blood flow.[57]

Acupuncture can influence hormonal functions

Many women visit our clinic for hormonal issues including follicle-stimulating hormone (FSH), luteinizing hormone (LH), estrogen, progesterone, prolactin, anti-mullerian hormone (AMH) and thyroid hormones. Acupuncture has been suggested as a valuable alternative therapy for female infertility due to hormone disorders.[58] For example, studies have shown improvement of reproductive hormone secretion patterns in women with PCOS.[59]

Acupuncture can also help adjust irregular menstrual cycles, because it influences the hormonal regulation centers in your brain and autonomic nervous system such as the hypothalamic-pituitary-ovarian/gonadal (HPG) axis and hypothalamic-pituitary-adrenal (HPA) axis.[60]

If you have stopped taking birth control pills, you may have an irregular cycle or a lack of period (amenorrhea). Acupuncture can help restore your cycle. The oral contraceptive pill prevents your body from making female hormones involved in ovulation and menstruation, because the pill artificially mimics your natural monthly fluctuation of hormones. When you stop taking the pill, it can take time for your body to return to a normal production of these hormones and generate a natural monthly cycle. Most women experience a return of regular ovulatory cycles soon after stopping the pill. However, if your period does not turn for several months, you may have post-pill amenorrhea. Acupuncture assists your natural hormone cycle by influencing the HPG axis (ovarian hormone feedback loops). Studies have also demonstrated positive effects of acupuncture on ovulation induction.[61]

Acupuncture and Egg Quality

If you have high FSH or low AMH levels or both, you are one of many patients who are struggling to conceive likely due to poor egg quality and low ovarian reserve. Unfortunately, it is a difficult condition to reverse because it is considered a part of the aging process. However, acupuncture can increase blood flow to your ovaries, which can help improve your ovarian function. Acupuncture cannot reverse the aging process but it is important to remember that there are two types of aging: chronological and biological. While everyone ages at the same speed chronologically, the biological aging process differs greatly among individuals. That is why each woman goes into menopause at a different time in her life. While it is generally true that the quality of a woman's eggs declines as she ages, the eggs of some women in their forties can be of excellent quality due to slow biological aging.

Progression of biological aging is mainly determined by genetic and lifestyle factors. The only factor you can change is lifestyle. Poor diet, smoking, stress, and insufficient sleep, accelerate cell damage and the biological aging process. While I have reservations in using the statement that acupuncture can reverse the aging process, I have had several cases in our clinic in which women over fifty, who were postmenopausal, began to have regular menstruation cycles after receiving acupuncture on a regular basis for general health. Practicing a healthy lifestyle in addition to regular acupuncture treatments will have a positive impact on your fertility.

Fertility Acupuncture Procedures

Fertility acupuncture points

More than 2,000 acupuncture points exist on the human body, connected by meridian channels. Currently, the World Health Organization recognizes 361.[62] The points located along meridian channels such as the spleen, liver, kidney, and bladder meridians, as well as the conception vessel, are particularly important for infertility. Some of the most well-known acupuncture points traditionally used for infertility are located on your low back, sacrum, lower abdomen, and legs. These regions are also considered very important from a nervous system perspective. It has been discovered that parts of your body's surface have a close neural association with a specific internal organ.[63]

Your reproductive organs are connected with your lumbar sacrum regions, so if you have conditions such as ovarian cysts, uterine fibroids or bad menstrual cramping, you may feel pain in your low abdomen and in your low back, hips and thighs. Based on experimental studies and traditional Chinese meridian theory, selecting traditional acupuncture points that are located within reproductive organ reflex areas can have a profound impact on reproductive organs. A series of laboratory studies on rats demonstrated that stimulating acupuncture points located within the reproductive reflex areas of low back and sacrum, significantly influenced ovarian and uterine blood flow.[64]

Many other acupuncture points traditionally used for fertility are located outside of the reproductive reflex areas, but they influence reproductive organs via other mechanisms. For example, I often stimulate the TE5 point, located near your wrist, with the SES acupuncture method (repetitive superficial acupuncture needling stimulation applied synchronically with your breathing).[65] This is typically done at the end of each acupuncture session, and is intended to optimize your reproductive and whole-body functions.

When and how often should you receive acupuncture?

You should receive acupuncture treatments on a regular basis, one to two times a week throughout your cycle, especially during an initial treatment period (the first two to three months) in order to correct any underlying imbalances. Regular acupuncture treatments can produce significant long-lasting benefits. Following the initial period, you may be advised to focus the treatment on a specific phase of your menstrual cycle.

Our fertility protocol[66] utilizes different acupuncture procedures depending on the phase of your menstrual cycle (during menstruation, pre-ovulation, ovulation/pre-implantation and pre-menstrual phases) in order to increase the therapeutic effect and safety of the treatment.

After the potential implantation period (usually six to nine days post-ovulation), it is important to consider the possibility of pregnancy and modify the acupuncture protocol accordingly. The treatment during the later part of the cycle (the phase four approach) is extremely gentle, intended to induce relaxation and minimize the release of harmful stress hormones, which can also help decrease unwanted uterine contractions. Our phase four approach is not only absolutely safe, but it also helps stabilize the implantation of the embryo. Therefore, I usually recommend that patients for whom implantation is a concern (especially those who have histories of recurrent early miscarriages) continue the treatment during their first trimester.

What is Moxibustion?

The term moxibustion comes from the Japanese "mogusa" meaning the herb moxa (Artemisia princeps, commonly called Japanese mugwort) and the Latin "bustion" meaning burning. It is a form of thermal therapy that involves burning the moxa over acupuncture points,[67] either by direct or indirect moxibustion. Indirect moxibustion, commonly used today, provides thermal stimulation without direct contact between the burning moxa and the skin's surface.[68]

Moxibustion is integral to the original concept of acupuncture and has been used with acupuncture to treat a variety of diseases throughout Asia for thousands of years. However, it is virtually ignored by many acupuncturists in Western countries and few people have tried it. I consider moxibustion vital for many fertility-related health concerns. Many women who have difficulty conceiving have symptoms of cold hands and feet even in the summertime, and sufficient blood flow to their reproductive organs is often compromised. The heat stimulation applied on selected acupuncture points helps to increase blood circulation to the uterus and pelvic area. It also induces a deep relaxation response that aids fertility.

From a physiological perspective, acupuncture and moxibustion work differently. While acupuncture induces a response through action on your nervous system, moxibustion acts more directly on your circulatory or immune system. Acupuncture used in conjunction with moxibustion profoundly enhances each modality's effects and potential benefits.

Moxibustion is different from other types of heating therapy such as the heat lamp and heating pad. Indirect moxibustion provides mild soothing heat to specific acupuncture points, whereas the heat lamp and heating pad warm up a much wider area or region of your body. Unlike a sauna or hot tub, moxibustion does not cause you to sweat or elevate your core body temperature.

Acupuncture and Assisted Reproductive Technologies

Many patients visit acupuncturists while receiving medical fertility treatments such as IUI or IVF. Acupuncture in conjunction with such medical treatments may help increase not only the chance of conception, but also pain relief during oocyte (egg) retrieval.[69] It can also help manage stress and improve the quality of life of patients undergoing IVF.[70]

When should I start acupuncture and how often should I receive treatment?

We often recommend that you start acupuncture treatment at least one to two months prior to the commencement of the IVF cycle and that you continue one to two times a week until the day of the transfer. This acupuncture IVF schedule is consistent with the recommendation and protocols used by American[71] and Japanese[72] advanced reproductive medicine centers. However, it is never too late to start acupuncture.

While you would likely obtain more cumulative benefits from the treatment by starting earlier, it would still help to receive acupuncture in any phase of the IVF cycle. At our clinic, many women continue their treatments after the transfer because they find it so relaxing and calming, and because it helps decrease their anxiety while waiting for pregnancy test results. Our post-transfer acupuncture protocol is similar to our gentle phase four approach used during the pre-menstrual phase.

Acupuncture protocol used in German study

In April 2002, German researchers reported that they had increased the success rate by nearly 50 percent in women undergoing IVF using acupuncture[73]. The study was highly publicized, so the German acupuncture protocol quickly became a "gold standard" during an IVF cycle and has been used by many acupuncturists. However, other investigators[74] and the original German group[75] failed to replicate their findings. Systematic review studies that analyzed the effectiveness of German protocol acupuncture with IVF pregnancy rates showed conflicting results[76]. I have never used the German protocol, and many acupuncturists current with the latest research no longer follow it.

Herbal Medicine and Fertility

Kampo medicine[77] is a traditional Japanese therapeutic system, primarily derived from the classical Chinese medicine that came to Japan in the fifth and sixth centuries. Kampo includes most of the traditional Chinese medicine (TCM) modalities including acupuncture, moxibustion, diet, and herbal medicine.

A variety of herbs have traditionally been used to improve the health of reproductive organs.[78] In recent years, Kampo and TCM formulas have been studied for various reproductive and gynecological applications.[79] Accordingly, a growing number of Japanese physicians and specialists have been prescribing Kampo formulations on a routine basis for their patients.

The word "herb" usually refers to a medicinal or aromatic plant.[80] In Chinese herbal medicine, however, herbal medicines are not only derived from plants, fruits or trees but also from rocks, shells, and different parts of animals, such as their skin, bones, or organs. Thus, herbal medicine is different from purely botanical medicine. The majority of Kampo and TCM medicines, however, are botanicals derived from plant-based herbs grown in Europe and in other parts of the world.

There is a distinct difference in usage of herbs by Western and Eastern herbalists. Western herbalists operate methodically, and usually consider a single herb for each condition, such as red raspberry leaf tea for the uterine lining or vitex (chaste berry) extract for regulating the menstrual cycle.

Practitioners of Kampo or TCM will often use a variety of herbs at one time in different combinations. They use a number of classical herbal formulas, comprised of five to ten or more different herbs, in specific combinations that have been used for thousands of years.

Some of the commonly prescribed herbal formulas for fertility patients include herbs that help improve blood circulation, calm the nervous system, and aid digestion. The traditional belief has been that through combining different herbs, both the enhancement of the effects provided by certain herbs as well as the neutralization of the negative effects of others, including toxicity, can be achieved.

Determining an appropriate Kampo and TCM formula requires a *sho* or *pattern*. Sho is very different from Western diagnosis. Women with the same health concern can reflecta different sho and be prescribed different Kampo or TCM prescriptions. Conversely, the same Kampo or TCM formulas may be used on women with different health issues, if they reflect the same sho. Women with endometriosis may be prescribed different herbal formulas if their sho is different, whereas, women who are having a short cycle or a long cycle may be prescribed the same formula if they have the same sho. Each woman's sho is determined within the context of an Eastern view of human anatomy, physiology, pathology, and clinical assessments.

Tongue observation is one of the core components of the assessments. Traditionally, the characteristics of your tongue reveal your underlying illness or imbalances. A recent study suggested that how the back part of your tongue looks (sublingual veins), could have a significant correlation with your menstrual symptoms.[81] Kampo and TCM practitioners make extensive use of terms such as yin/yang, exterior/ interior, cold/heat, and vacuity/repletion in determining the nature of your illness, and then may prescribe different herbal formulas depending on the phase of your menstrual cycle.

Traditional East Asian Medicine Dietary Approach to Fertility

Proper diet is extremely important for recovery from many illnesses, as well as for the maintenance of good health. In fact, it is so important that diet is an integral part of traditional East Asian medicine—as food therapy. In Kampo, it is called *shokuyou*, and in TCM, this practice is known as *shi liao*.

In Western nutrition, the individual approach will primarily focus on analyzing the nutritional values of each portion or meal. Kampo and TCM, by contrast, emphasize the characteristics of whole foods, because they believe that every food has specific thermal characteristics, known as thermal nature. Foods can be hot, warm, neutral, cool or cold. Kampo practitioners consider these characteristics as elements that will affect an individual's constitution. For example, a Western nutritionist may recommend a salad containing ingredients like lettuce, tomatoes, and oranges, as a source of vitamins, to a broad range of people. According to the thermal nature of foods in Kampo, however, these foods are considered cold or cool. The over-consumption of such vegetables and fruits is not recommended for certain groups of individuals (e.g., cold/spleen vacuity types).

Conversely, if someone is expressing *heat* constitutional patterns, they may be encouraged to eat those foods that are cold or cool in nature. Ginger provides another interesting contrast. From a Western nutrition analysis point of view, ginger is a source of potassium. In Kampo, ginger is extremely valuable as both an herb and a medicinal food. The warming effect of ginger is highly valuable for people with a *cold* constitution, and when combined with other herbs, ginger enhances the effects of other warming herbs and decreases the undesirable side effects of herbs with cooling natures.

The main tenet of the Kampo diet is the concept of balancing the *yin* (cold) and the *yang* (warm). Traditional East Asian medicine practitioners provide general dietary guidelines based on each person's constitutional pattern. The main diagnostic criteria include signs of repletion/vacuity, heat/cold, and dampness/dryness. It is extremely important that the digestive tract always be kept warm, especially in vacuity and cold-type individuals.

Many women who have difficulty conceiving are categorized as having a yin constitution. In the Kampo point of view, women with a yin constitution who regularly consume large amounts of foods and drinks that cool down their internal organs could be interfering with the proper functioning of their reproductive systems.

In my experience as a resident of Canada, I have noticed that many people, especially young females, overeat raw vegetable salads and fruits. Eating a large bowl of vegetable salad may be good for replete body types that tend to accumulate *heat* (typically, individuals with such constitutions tend to develop heart disease, high cholesterol, high blood pressure, diabetes, and stroke). On the other hand, for individuals with other constitutional types, such as *vacuity* with *cold* (many infertility patients fit into this category), consuming large amounts of raw vegetables and fruits may not be beneficial.

Women with a yin constitution should consume more yang foods and minimize their intake of foods with a yin nature; women with a yang constitution should eat more yin foods and decrease their intake of foods with a yang nature. This balance is integral to understanding the Kampo and TCM diet.

Stress and infertility

The journey to conception can be physically and emotionally stressful for many women due to fear of failure or social pressure, sometimes combined with self-esteem issues. However, it is important to learn to reduce and manage stress, as studies indicate a relationship between stress and infertility[82] and stress and unsuccessful IVF.[83] Medical tests and treatments for infertility are also major sources of stress for many women who are having difficulty conceiving.[84]

Stress can have such a negative impact on fertility because stress hormones such as catecholamines (adrenalin, noradrenalin, and dopamine) and the hypothalamic-pituitary-adrenal axis (our central stress response system) interact with hormones that are responsible for normal ovulatory cycles (i.e., GnRH, prolactin, LH, and FSH).[85] Some hormones that are released during times of stress can cause the uterus to contract and/or negatively interact with immune cells, both of which will interfere with proper implantation.[86]

How acupuncture can assist you to combat stress

Although having a bunch of needles inserted under your skin may not sound like a way to relax, acupuncture has frequently and successfully been used for stress-related disorders.[87] Many people start snoozing immediately after a few needles are inserted. That is because of the effects of acupuncture on your autonomic nervous system. Your autonomic nervous system is divided into two parts: the parasympathetic system (which allows your body to relax and aids your digestion and other important internal body functions) and the sympathetic system (which responds to high stress situations by causing heart pounding, dry mouth, cold hands, or increased sweating).

Acupuncture inhibits the sympathetic and activates the parasympathetic, in most cases both at the same time, to slow your heart rate and provide a relaxation effect. This unique acupuncture response has been confirmed numerous times clinically and by experimental studies.[88]

I have been utilizing the treatment method called Acupuncture and Sound Assisted Autonomic Modulation technique, which is a combination of acupuncture and a particular slow breathing exercise with sound prompts.[89] You breathe in a specific rhythm while lying on the table with acupuncture needles inserted, in order to modulate and optimize your autonomic nervous system and enhance your innate healing abilities.

In Closing

The main concept of acupuncture and traditional East Asian medicine is addressing the whole body and mind to help create the most desirable physical and mental conditions for conception.

During your session, your acupuncturist will gently support your body and nudge it towards balance and harmony. Your mind will restore its positive attitude towards healing, and your body will open its channels for a smooth flow of energy, releasing negative stagnation and letting the unobstructed blood flow harmonize the function of your organs.

Whether you would like to try acupuncture and traditional East Asian medicine to become pregnant naturally, use it as complementary treatment with IVF, or simply want to relax and de-stress between your fertility specialist's appointments, your acupuncturist can assist you. However, the ultimate creator and traveler on this journey is YOU. Best Wishes.

---

[48] G. Maciocia, *Obstetrics and Gynecology in Chinese Medicine* (New York: Churchill Livingstone, 1998).
[49] A. Burke et al., "Acupuncture Use in the United States: findings from the National Health Interview Survey," *Journal of Alternative and Complementary Medicine* 12, no. 7 (September 2006): 639-648.
[50] W.E. Paulus et al., "Influence of Acupuncture on the Pregnancy Rate in Patients Who Undergo Assisted Reproduction Therapy," *Fertility and Sterility* 77, no. 4 (April 2002): 721-724.
[51] S. Uchida et al., "Ovarian Blood Flow is Reflexively Regulated by Mechanical Afferent Stimulation of a Hindlimb in Nonpregnant Anesthetized Rats," *Autonomic Neuroscience* 106, no. 2 (July 31, 2003): 91-97; H. Hotta et al., "Uterine Contractility and Blood Flow are Reflexively Regulated by Cutaneous Afferent Stimulation in Anesthetized Rats," *Journal of the Autonomic Nervous System* 75, no. 1 (January 15,

1999): 23-31; E. Stener-Victorin et al., "Reduction of Blood Flow Impedance in the Uterine Arteries of Infertile Women with Electro-Acupuncture," *Human Reproduction* 11, no. 6 (June 1996): 1314-1317.

[52] S. Emmons and P. Patton, "Acupuncture Treatment for Infertile Women Undergoing Intracytoplasmic Sperm Injection," *Medical Acupuncture: A Journal for Physicians by Physicians* 12, no. 2 (2000).

[53] Hotta et al., "Uterine Contractility and Blood Flow," 23-31; Stener-Victorin et al., "Reduction of Blood Flow Impedance," 1314-1317.

[54] H. Fu et al., "Acupuncture on the Endometrial Morphology, the Serum Estradiol and Progesterone Levels, and the Expression of Endometrial Leukaemia-inhibitor Factor and Osteopontin in Rats," *Evidence-based Complementary and Alternative Medicine* 2011, Article ID 606514; Z. Shuai et al., "Effect of Transcutaneous Electrical Acupuncture Point Stimulation on Endometrial Receptivity in Women Undergoing Frozen-Thawed Embryo Transfer: a Single-Blind Prospective Randomised Controlled Trial," *Acupuncture Medicine* (October 10, 2014).

[55] M. Rubinstein et al., "Low-dose Aspirin Treatment Improves Ovarian Responsiveness, Uterine and Ovarian Blood Flow Velocity, Implantation, and Pregnancy Rates in Patients Undergoing In Vitro Fertilization: a Prospective, Randomized, Double-Blind Placebo-Controlled Assay," *Fertility and Sterility* 71, no. 5 (May 1999): 825-829.

[56] G. Sher and J.D. Fisch, "Vaginal Sildenafil (Viagra): a Preliminary Report of a Novel Method to Improve Uterine Artery Blood Flow and Endometrial Development in Patients Undergoing IVF," *Human Reproduction* 15, no. 4 (April 2000): 806-809.

[57] A. Sato et al., "Calcitonin Gene-Related Peptide Produces Skeletal Muscle Vasodilation Following Antidromic Stimulation of Unmyelinated Afferents in the Dorsal Root in Rats," *Neuroscience Letters*, 283, no. 2 (April 7, 2000): 137-140.

[58] I. Gerhard and F. Postneek, "Auricular Acupuncture in the Treatment of Female Infertility," Gynecological Endocrinology 6, no. 3 (September 1992): 171-181.

[59] 59 E. Stener-Victorin et al., "Effects of Electro-Acupuncture on Anovulation in Women with Polycystic Ovary Syndrome," *Acta Obstetricia et Gynecologica Scandinavica* 79, no. 3 (March 2000): 180-188; J. Johansson et al., "Acupuncture for Ovulation Induction in Polycystic Ovary Syndrome: a Randomized Controlled Trial," *American Journal of Physiology, Endocrinology and Metabolism* 304, no. 9 (May 1, 2013): E934-943.

[60] E. Stener-Victorin et al., "Effects of Electro-Acupuncture on Corticotropin-Releasing Factor in Rats With Experimentally-Induced Polycystic Ovaries," *Neuropeptides* 35, no. 5-6 (October- December 2001): 227-231.

[61] Stener-Victorin et al., "Effects of Electro-Acupuncture on Anovulation," 180-188; Johansson et al., "Acupuncture for Ovulation Induction," E934-943; B.Y. Chen and J. Yu, "Relationship Between Blood Radioimmunoreactive Beta-Endorphin and Hand Skin Temperature During the Electro-Acupuncture Induction of Ovulation," *Acupuncture and Electrotherapeutics Research* 16, no. 1 -2 (1991): 1-5; X. Mo et al., "Clinical Studies on the Mechanism for Acupuncture Stimulation of Ovulation," *Journal of Traditional Chinese Medicine* 13, no. 2 (June 1993): 115-119.

[62] *World Health Organization Standard Acupuncture Nomenclature*, 2nd ed. (Manila: World Health Organization, 1993).
[63] J.J. Bonica, "Applied Anatomy Relevant to Pain," in *The Management of Pain*, vol. 1, 2nd ed., ed. J.J. Bonica (Philadelphia: Lea & Febiger, 1990), 133-158.
[64] Uchida et al., "Ovarian Blood Flow," 91-97; Hotta et al., "Uterine Contractility and Blood Flow," 23-31.
[65] H. Mori et al., "Is There Any Difference in Human Pupillary Reaction When Different Acupuncture Points Are Stimulated?" *Acupuncture in Medicine* 28, no. 1 (March 2010): 21-24; K. Nishijo et al., "Scientific Approach for Acupuncture," *Journal of the Japan Society of Acupuncture and Moxibustion* 45, no. 3 (1995): 177-191; T.H. Tanaka, G. Leisman, and K. Nishijo, "The Physiological Responses Induced by Superficial Acupuncture: a Comparative Study of Acupuncture Stimulation During Exhalation Phase and Continuous Stimulation," *International Journal of Neuroscience* 90, no. 1-2 (June 1997): 45-58.
[66] T.H. Tanaka, "Fertility Difficulties Treated by Acupuncture: Analysis of 76 Pregnancy Cases," The 20th Year Anniversary WFAS International Acupuncture Congress (Beijing, China: 2007).
[67] L. Gwei-Djen and J. Needham, "Moxibustion," in *Celestial Lancets: A History and Rationale of Acupuncture and Moxa* (London: Cambridge University Press, 1980), 170-184.
[68] Mori et al., "One-Point and Three-Point Indirect Moxibustion Stimulation," 27-31.
[69] S.M. Sator-Katzenschlager et al., "Auricular Electro-Acupuncture as an Additional Perioperative Analgesic Method During Oocyte Aspiration in IVF Treatment," *Human Reproduction* 21, no. 8 (August 2006): 2114-2120; E. Stener-Victorin et al., "A Prospective Randomized Study of Electro-Acupuncture Versus Alfentanil as Anaesthesia During Oocyte Aspiration in In Vitro Fertilization," Human Reproduction 14, no. 10 (October 1999): 2480-2484; P. Humaidan and E. Stener-Victorin, "Pain Relief During Oocyte Retrieval With a New Short Duration Electro-Acupuncture Technique: An Alternative to Conventional Analgesic Methods," *Human Reproduction* 19, no. 6 (June 2004): 1367-1372.
[70] B.J. Anderson et al., "In Vitro Fertilization and Acupuncture: Clinical Efficacy and Mechanistic Basis," *Alternative Therapies in Health and Medicine* 13, no. 3 (May-June 2007): 38-48; A.L. Gejervall et al., "Electro-Acupuncture Versus Conventional Analgesia: A Comparison of Pain Levels During Oocyte Aspiration and Patients' Experiences of Well-Being After Surgery," *Human Reproduction* 20, no. 3 (March 2005): 728-735.
[71] P.C. Magarelli, D.K. Cridennda, and M. Cohen, "Changes in Serum Cortisol and Prolactin Associated with Acupuncture During Controlled Ovarian Hyperstimulation in Women Undergoing In Vitro Fertilization-Embryo Transfer Treatment," *Fertility and Sterility* 92, no. 6 (December 2009): 1870-1879.
[72] H. Suzuki, "Infertility and Acupuncture Treatment," *The Japanese Journal of Acupuncture and Moxibustion Therapies* 65, no. 6 (2006).
[73] Paulus et al., "Influence of Acupuncture on the Pregnancy Rate," 721-724.
[74] C. Smith, M. Coyle, and R.J. Norman, "Influence of Acupuncture Stimulation on Pregnancy Rates for Women Undergoing Embryo Transfer," *Fertility and Sterility* 85,

no. 5 (May 2006): 1352-1358; A.D. Domar et al., "The Impact of Acupuncture on In Vitro Fertilization Outcome," *Fertility and Sterility* 91, no. 3 (March 2009): 723-726; D. Andersen et al., "Acupuncture on the Day of Embryo Transfer: A Randomized Controlled Trial of 635 Patients," *Reproductive Biomedicine Online* 21, no. 3 (September 2010): 366-372; M. Benson, K. Elkind-Hirsch, and A. Theall, "Impact of Acupuncture Before and After Embryo Transfer on the Outcome of In Vitro Fertilization Cycle: A Prospective Single Blind Randomized Study," *Fertility and Sterility* 86 (2006): 583-587; I. Moy et al., "Randomized Controlled Trial: Effects of Acupuncture on Pregnancy Rates in Women Undergoing In Vitro Fertilization," *Fertility and Sterility* 95, no. 2 (February 2011): 583-587.

[75] W.E. Paulus et al., "Placebo-Controlled Trial of Acupuncture Effects in Assisted Reproductive Therapy," (paper, Abstract of the 19th Annual Meeting of the ESHRE, Madrid, Spain, 2003).

[76] S.K. Sunkara et al., "Acupuncture and In Vitro Fertilization: Updated Meta-Analysis," *Human Reproduction* 24, no. 8 (August 2009): 2047-2048; T. El-Toukhy et al., "A Systematic Review and Meta-Analysis of Acupuncture in In Vitro Fertilisation," *BJOG: An International Journal of Obstetrics and Gynaecology* 115, no. 10 (September 2008): 1203-1213; E. Manheimer et al., "Effects of Acupuncture on Rates of Pregnancy and Live Birth Among Women Undergoing In Vitro Fertilisation: Systematic Review and Meta-Analysis," BMJ 336, no. 7643 (March 8, 2008): 545-549.

[77] Kampo, https://kampo.ca.

[78] Maciocia, *Obstetrics and Gynecology*.

[79] N. Kotani et al., "Analgesic Effect of a Herbal Medicine for Treatment of Primary Dysmenorrhea—A Double-Blind Study," *The American Journal of Chinese Medicine* 25, no. 2 (1997): 205-212; A. Oya et al., "Clinical Efficacy of Kampo Medicine (Japanese traditional herbal medicine) in the Treatment of Primary Dysmenorrhea," *The Journal of Obstetrics and Gynaecology Research* 34, no. 5 (October 2008): 898-908; T. Tanaka, "A Novel Anti-Dysmenorrhea Therapy with Cyclic Administration of Two Japanese Herbal Medicines," Clinical and Experimental Obstetrics & Gynecology 30, no. 2-3 (2003): 95-98; T. Ushiroyama et al., "Unkei-To for Correcting Luteal Phase Defects," *The Journal of Reproductive Medicine* 48, no. 9 (September 2003): 729-734; T. Ushiroyama et al., "Effects of Unkei-To, an Herbal Medicine, on Endocrine Function and Ovulation in Women with High Basal Levels of Luteinizing Hormone Secretion," The Journal of Reproductive Medicine 46, no. 5 (May 2001): 451-456; and K. Yamada and S. Kanba, "Effectiveness of Kamishoyosan for Premenstrual Dysphoric Disorder: Open-Labeled Pilot Study," *Psychiatry and Clinical Neurosciences* 61, no. 3 (June 2007): 323-325.

[80] L. Winslow and D. Kroll, "Herbs as Medicines," *Archives of Internal Medicine* 158, no. 20 (1998): 2192-2199.

[81] T.H. Tanaka, "Tongue Diagnosis: Relationship Between Sublingual Tongue Morphology in Three Tongue Protrusion Angles and Menstrual Clinical Symptoms," *Journal of Integrative Medicine* 13, no. 4 (July 2015): 248-256.

[82] G.P. Chrousos, D.J. Torpy and P.W. Gold, "Interactions Between the Hypothalamic-Pituitary-Adrenal Axis and the Female Reproductive System: Clinical Implications,"

Annals of Internal Medicine 129, no. 3 (August 1, 1998): 229-240; H. Matsubayashi et al., "Spontaneous Conception in a 50-Year-Old Woman After Giving Up In Vitro Fertilization (IVF) Treatments: Involvement of the Psychological Relief in Successful Pregnancy," *Tokai Journal of Experimental and Clinical Medicine* 28, no. 1 (April 2003): 9-15.

[83] A. Eugster and A.J. Vingerhoets, "Psychological Aspects of In Vitro Fertilization: A Review," *Social Science and Medicine* 48, no. 5 (March 1999): 575-589; A. Gallinelli et al., "Immunological Changes and Stress Are Associated with Different Implantation Rates in Patients Undergoing In Vitro Fertilization-Embryo Transfer," *Fertility and Sterility* 76, no. 1 (July 2001): 85-91; J.M. Smeenk et al., "Stress and Outcome Success in IVF: The Role of Self-Reports and Endocrine Variables," *Human Reproduction* (January 21, 2005).

[84] C.R. Harlow et al., "Stress and Stress-Related Hormones During In-Vitro Fertilization Treatment, " *Human Reproduction* 11, no. 2 (February 1996): 274-279; M.S. Kupka et al., "Stress Relief After Infertility Treatment—Spontaneous Conception, Adoption and Psychological Counseling," *European Journal of Obstetrics & Gynecology and Reproductive Biology* 110, no. 2 (October 10, 2003): 190-195; and J.G. Schenker, D. Meirow, and E. Schenker, "Stress and Human Reproduction," *European Journal of Obstetrics & Gynecology and Reproductive Biology* 45, no. 1 (June 16, 1992): 1-8.

[85] Schenker, Meirow, and Schenker, "Stress and Human Reproduction," 1-8.

[86] Gallinelli et al.,"Immunological Changes and Stress," 85-91; G.Sher, V. Davis and J. Stoess, "*In Vitro Fertilization*," (New York: Facts on File, 1998).

[87] Y.D. Kim et al., "Acupuncture for Posttraumatic Stress Disorder: A Systematic Review of Randomized Controlled Trials and Prospective Clinical Trials," *Evidence-Based Complementary Alternative Medicine* Article ID 615857 (2013); K. Pilkington et al., "Acupuncture for Anxiety and Anxiety Disorders—A Systematic Literature Review," Acupuncture Medicine 25, no. 1-2 (June 2007): 1-10.

[88] T.H. Tanaka, "The Possibilities for Optimizing Acupuncture Treatment Results Through Synchronization with Somatic State: Examination of Autonomic Response to Superficial Needling During Exhalation," *American Journal of Acupuncture* 24, no. 4 (1996): 233-239; K. Nishijo et al., "Decreased Heart Rate by Acupuncture Stimulation in Humans via Facilitation of Cardiac Vagal Activity and Suppression of Cardiac Sympathetic Nerve," Neuroscience Letters 227, no. 3 (May 23, 1997): 165-168; and H. Mori et al., "Effects of Acupuncture Treatment on Natural Killer Cell Activity, Pulse Rate, and Pain Reduction for Older Adults: An Uncontrolled, Observational Study," *Journal of Integrative Medicine* 11, no. 2 (March 2013): 101-105.

[89] T.H. Tanaka, "Enhancement of Acupuncture Effects with Auditory Assisted Slow Breathing,"(paper, WHO Congress on Traditional Medicine, Bejing, China, 2008); T.H. Tanaka, "Potentiating the Autonomic Effects of Acupuncture by Proactive Use of Respiration," (paper, ICMART XIII World Congress, Budapest, Hungary, 2008).

Chapter 3: Mind-Body Awareness

My Healing Journey

I first learned about my coach after I found a stop smoking hypnosis special that she was advertising. I had purchased it for my husband in hopes that he would be open to giving it a try. As it turned out, he wasn't, so instead of losing my purchase I phoned her and asked if she offered any other type of counseling or hypnosis. I was embarking on a path of self-focus and healing, as I had experienced a miscarriage a few months before. She said she could help me achieve some of my personal goals, such as maintaining a commitment to a healthier lifestyle (i.e., exercise and a healthy diet). In my life, it had been a challenge to follow through in a number of areas such as eating healthy, exercising, education, and even close relationships.

Prior to our first meeting, my coach had me complete a very detailed questionnaire that really had me dig deep and begin to identify some main areas where I wanted to see change.

My main challenges were not feeling good enough, not feeling heard, fearing death, not feeling respected, being critical of myself, avoiding confrontations, and feeling sadness, regret, hurt, guilt, and anxiousness surrounding my miscarriage and my continued desire to have another child.

My main goals were to have another child, spend more quality time with my husband and our two children, maintain my career, improve my relationship and intimacy with my husband, be healthier and exercise regularly, start rock climbing again, consistently go to yoga and for walks, and become a better planner. Quite a list!

During our first meeting, we worked to identify and clear the root emotion behind many of my challenges. One of these roots—or as my coach refers to them, rocks—was abandonment and unworthiness. I left our meeting feeling encouraged that I was on the right path for me in this moment in my life. My coach was like a new old friend; I instantly felt comfortable with her and found her to be very caring and supportive, with a straightforward approach that kept me focused and on track.

I experienced a second miscarriage a few days before our second meeting. The only positive thing I could take from my miscarriage was that it was fast and without complications. During our meeting, my coach and I identified my immediate concerns: I wanted to have another child but I felt my husband was not fully committed to my desire, so I felt disrespected and not heard or supported. I felt life was passing me by and I didn't want to wait any longer. Deep down, I knew that this process of wanting another baby had put me in a limbo state where I was not fully engaged with my existing beautiful family.

She helped me rebalance and clear the emotions of anger and sadness through Time Line Therapy® and Neuro-Linguistic Programming (NLP). I remember doubting the effectiveness of this therapy. However, I found when I "checked in" to see if I could feel any pain and anger, I realized to my amazement that I could remember the events without reliving the feeling of the emotion. I had healing!

One take away from this meeting was that I needed to do something for myself. I have always wanted to own and learn to play a steel string guitar. I had an old classical one from my childhood that I could strum on a little, but I felt compelled to fulfill my dream of learning to play a steel string. So I went out and bought one!

My coach and I met again a couple of weeks later. I had purchased my new guitar and I was feeling much better about my relationship with my husband. My coach had given me some homework to complete after our last session: my husband and I were to identify our preferred way of showing love to each other by completing the short exercise in *The Five Love Languages: The Secret to Love That Lasts*, by Gary Chapman. Both my hubby and I worked through this exercise and it helped us realize some of the imbalances between what we were giving and receiving, and what we needed and wanted from each other. Once again, my coach used Time Line Therapy™ and NLP to rebalance and clear more root emotions of fear, doubt, distrust, unworthiness, hurt, and guilt. I remember this was a pretty heavy session, and as we wrapped up that evening. I knew we were beginning to lay the groundwork for a new direction for my thoughts and emotions. I trusted that this path would serve me better than the counterproductive ones I had been using.

Two weeks later, we reviewed my journaling efforts for the activity called, "Goal, Purpose, Need to Do." It was meant to set awareness and intention into each new day by having me physically put pen to paper and document a goal, a direction, and a reason why. I found that this gave me a new and positive focus for the day. It helped me look outside of my own bubble of yearning for a baby and yearning for other changes that were outside my power. It put the focus on improving the world one or two steps outside myself.

Some of my revelations from this exercise were about my relationship with my sister as well as my husband, so my coach and I discussed setting boundaries. In the past, I was a pleaser, so much so that I would lose my own voice, putting my wants, needs, thoughts, and ideas on the back burner. This made me feel disregarded and hurt. We worked through rebalancing and clearing resentment, not feeling respected, fear, and not feeling heard. And we did a short exercise to help me feel excitement again.

We also discussed wealth and material items. I have always wanted just enough money to allow for freedom and a good quality of life, and I have never visualized or expected to have more than that. I believe too much material stuff can get in the way of loving and quality communication and time spent together. We discovered that deep down, money made me feel lonely, insecure, and untrusting. We were successful in changing that limiting belief to trusting.

A month later, I was feeling a bit discouraged and sensed I had much more work to do. I had succeeded in putting regular exercise back into my life. However, some of the old challenges still existed between my husband and I, and I was having issues with an individual at work. My coach and I reviewed the importance of planning for things such as meals and date night with my husband, and we discussed which boundaries I needed to set for my workplace.

Over our next few sessions, it was evident that I still had my old habits of lack of follow through, and I was not holding up my end of the bargain when it came to boundary enforcement. A number of things seemed to be sliding and we worked on clearing the limiting belief of "not important." Soon afterwards, I went on a vacation to spend some time with my family and when I returned, I discovered I was pregnant.

I knew I still had more work to do, but I felt like I was in a better place for this pregnancy to be a strong and healthy one. I was so excited to be pregnant, and on the right track that I was certain I would immerse myself in any activity needed over the next six months to get to that ultimate place of achievement. Then I miscarried at nine weeks for the third time in twelve consecutive months. This miscarriage was the roughest yet and it took many hospital visits over many weeks before everything cleared naturally.

I took an extended leave from work to focus on my physical healing. This coincided with my girls returning to school that fall and I was able to be there with them. I focused on being thankful for the children I had and truly cherished this extra time with them. I was also able to gain the clear perspective that I needed to change my work situation. A few weeks later, I was blessed with a layoff notice—due to downsizing—and finished my employment with that company.

One of my greatest regrets over the past few years has been that I've missed out on precious time with my young girls. Since my husband was starting a new business, we had agreed that I would be the one working outside our home. But having my husband there, taking our girls to and from school and being there for them when I couldn't during the day, made me feel resentful and cheated. I was the one who was supposed to be with them—this was not our agreed-to plan. So now that I had been let go, I felt it was my turn. For the next few months, I threw myself into my girls and just enjoyed every bit I could. I also spent time understanding my husband's business, showing an interest, and even beginning to support his venture, probably for the first time ever. This brought us closer together than we had been in years.

While our girls were in school, I also took time to start my own business just to see if I could make a go of it. I gave myself three months and I was very clear as to what I was willing to put in, so as not to take away from my time with the girls. At the end of the three months, I felt good about my experience and decided self-employment was not for me. My husband's business was beginning to take a more positive direction and I made peace with the idea that I would return to work, however, not just for any old job; I had my eye on a very specific role and hoped I would not have to settle for less.

Reflecting on my old habit of "lack of follow through," I had never finished my education in business and human resources (HR), and always wanted to work in an HR department, but didn't feel good enough to land a corporate role. Well, "not good enough" went right out the window when I landed an HR specialist six-month contract the following spring. It felt like such an accomplishment; I was excited to go back to work!

This new position was amazing in almost every way and I thoroughly enjoyed going to work each day. During my first six- month contract term, a few things happened: I felt happy, I felt I was on the right track, I still wanted another baby—and I began to have a new health concern. I was not pregnant; however, my breasts became enlarged and very sore. I met with doctors, specialists, and a naturopath and we could not figure out the cause, but thankfully nothing showed up on any of the tests. I was certainly relieved, but the experience was unnerving.

I told my coach that I felt having a third child would bring me a kind of closure for all the pain I had experienced through the miscarriages. Part of me wanted my girls to experience a baby in the house and I wanted a chance for a "do over." My two girls are close in age, so when they were small, I was in an exhaustion haze and maybe didn't cherish as many of those little precious moments as I could have. I dreamed about nurturing another baby with my new self and soaking in every moment of it, but I knew my body needed a rest.

I was really hoping my company would hire me full time after my first contract; however, they did re-sign me for another six months early that fall. Though slightly discouraged, I was still very happy to continue in the hopes a full-time role would be in my future. During this time, I realized I was coming to a place of peace and acceptance—maybe, just maybe, I was not meant to have another baby. My breast symptoms had begun to subside and I was feeling more balanced than I had in a very long time. I had a beautiful family and this acceptance began to settle in just in time for me to experience a new pregnancy!

I was in utter shock to learn I was pregnant—we had only had intercourse one time that month and it was not the optimal time! I actually thought that my period was late due to possible early menopause! Well, there was no question in my mind that this was a miracle, a miracle baby. I was super nervous, more nervous than normal for me during the first trimester, but once I entered into the second trimester the nervousness began to subside. I began to release much of the fear and embrace the joy of a growing baby inside me.

And here we are today with three beautiful and healthy girls. I have a job I love, which allows me to have precious time with my babies before and after school, my husband and I continue to work on our relationship with growing success, and his business is still moving in a positive direction!

Mind-Body Awareness: The Difference that Makes the Difference in Results;

by Glenda Johnson

My intention for writing this chapter on the mind-body-spirit connection is that you may feel inspired and hear information said in a different way that will make sense to you when you see it on the written page. Maybe you will have awareness, some ahas, gain an understanding, realize some basic truths, and become inspired on your journey of self-discovery: realizing that everything happens for a reason, even those obstacles. I will show you how these life changes actually happen for your highest good. May you come away with the clarity of knowing that there are other choices and solutions out there, so you can know what to do next.

When I think about all the hundreds or maybe even thousands of modalities out there, including the traditional Western medicine system, and why you may get results with some of these and not with others, I've come to believe that it's the result of a few influential factors:

- where your coach currently is on their own journey of self-discovery, with their beliefs, their intentions and skill set;
- where you currently are on the emotional scale, where you want to go and whether you've "had enough yet";
- whether or not your coach holds their focus and intention that you are well already. It makes a difference when your coach believes that it's possible and holds your wellness within their mind's eye—it means you are already whole and have what you want.

When you first come to see me, you probably won't believe that the world you live in is loving and harmonious. Through the process, you will develop the willingness to look at your not-so-likeable qualities and do what it takes. You will be open to changing them and eventually believe, once again, that you deserve to love yourself and that you are not broken.

Ultimately, I believe that the difference that makes the real difference is utilizing the relationship between your mind, your body, and your spirit—

being aware. When I say spirit, I'm not talking about religion, I'm talking about your conscious awareness of what's going on inside and outside yourself— how you perceive the world, other people, and yourself.

I'm talking about accepting the basic principle that whatever you believe in your mind is reflected in your body. Your body cannot be experienced by itself; it can only be experienced through your mind, which is in every cell of your body (not just your brain) and is perceived through your consciousness and awareness.

Without your mind, you cannot experience the sensations that tell you about your body.

If you can understand that the experiences of your body are not happening in your body, but in your mind, then you can make changes within your mind that will ultimately affect your body.

You don't need to know the process for it to work. I include it here in case you are curious and want to know a little of the why and how.

So, if your body is only expressing what you hold or believe in your mind, then when you change your old beliefs, patterns, thoughts, and emotions, it will change what you see, feel, hear, and experience in your world.

Realize that it is your mind that has the power to create, whether health or disease. This is where the processes make the changes in your life.

This is where change and miracles happen.

Let me tell you how this works in your life within the context of coaching. You will only show up when "you've had enough"—when you're sick and tired of being sick and tired, or you're stuck and fearful of your future.

Any kind of serious event, illness, or setback presents a choice. You can feel sorry for yourself as a victim, have self-pity, be depressed, and feel despair, or you can see the setback as a challenge and an opportunity.

These events are usually a springboard to greater awareness. It takes maximum duress for you to stop and begin to question the reality of the things you've believed so far. Growth only happens when you're up against a major confrontation and the emotion has built to the point where you've had enough.

This is when you have the courage to do—to take action in order for your life to change. Like the "turning point" in the hockey game. As Winston Churchill said, "Success is not final, failure is not fatal: it is the courage to continue that counts."

You may come in filled with fear and anger, full of pride and *havingness*—looking outside yourself for *things* to fill you up. When you feel that your source of happiness and survival exists outside of yourself, it usually leads to a loss in your health because you have a "fear of loss" program running.

You don't really understand how you got to where you are. It's all about awareness. Carl Jung, a great psychologist, said, "You cannot change anything about yourself without becoming aware of it first."

As the brain is wired to always look for and attach to patterns, we look to replace the patterns/beliefs that don't serve us with life-giving ones. You need to have an open mind and be willing to let go of your negative energy patterns to face the truth about yourself. With that uncovering comes awareness and acceptance. Then you can turn the negative patterns that have been holding you back into positive ones by changing your limiting beliefs. Feeling compassion, forgiveness, and love for yourself and others has a curative and healing effect; it changes how you view and interpret life's events. I believe you magnetically attract people and circumstances to yourself based on your current beliefs.

Everybody is looking for *happiness* and for each of us it looks different. When it comes to infertility, of course, you're looking for a baby and the reasons vary greatly.

Will a baby make you happy or more fulfilled? Will it fill a void in your relationship or your career? Do you feel that you can't have your career and be a mother too? Will a baby fulfill your deep need for love and connection? Will it improve the quality of your life while you make a difference in another's?

No matter the issue, whether you want to have a baby, you're fed up with your career, or you're struggling with some chronic mental or physical health issue, there are lots of similarities in your unconscious programming. You may be feeling unworthy, invalidated, or inflated, judging others and yourself, always "winning" and being "right," full of guilt for things that you've done or didn't do, grieving your past, fearing your future, nursing your wounds, craving assurance, or seeking love instead of giving it.

If you believe that it isn't possible, then it isn't. What you believe, you see as evidence in your world. When you find the courage to open your mind and give something a go— *willingness*—then your beliefs can shift.

In the beginning, you may be like many people—without realizing it, you do not truly love yourself or your body and it affects your fertility.

Also, you must let go of your *attachment* to your current experience. You may do this right away and the shifts will be very noticeable in all areas of your life, or you may resist and take longer.

Through the coaching process, you will learn how to respond differently to events. The meaning you give them determines how you'll react to them. How you feel in that moment when an unexpected situation happens will affect your response.

Your emotions are one of the most powerful attributes that you own. They'll drive you to do something or not, and every decision you make is based on how you feel.

You rarely experience one emotion by itself. For example, if a major crisis arises and you feel guilt, that emotion will drag all the other destructive, negative ones with it.

You may blame yourself and ask, "Why didn't I do this?" or "Why didn't I see this before?" That is retrospective self- recrimination. Life might seem hopeless, you might feel like you'll never be happy again, and fear might come into the picture. You may become obsessed with changing it, begin to bargain with the higher power, or say it's somebody else's fault. That is emotional overwhelm.

With the simplest, leading edge, mind-body techniques and processes of neuro-linguistic programming (NLP), Time Line Therapy (TLT) ™, hypnotherapy, and Advanced Clearing Energetics (ACE) ™, we disconnect the fuse and pull the plug on your negative emotions. You gain new understanding and positive learning, and can look at past events with neutrality, which lets go of the energy of the upsets. The energy has been accumulating for your lifetime and now it has a way out. However, if you attempt to resist it your pain will increase due to your resistance of the experience.

We coaches say it's never about the story or the events; it's getting the excess feelings dealt with so that the events can be handled.

There were times when you may have felt that these problems were catastrophic, hopeless, unbearable, and insurmountable. Those issues would have been so simple to solve if you could have gotten the emotions out of the way.

Think about this: You determine what you do want by first identifying what you don't want. The better you feel about yourself, the more your life view changes.

David Hawkins explains this so well: "The willingness to *forgive* can move us into the willingness to be compassionate. Having compassion means the willingness to see the innocence within all things, which coincides with the willingness to forgive. Out of compassion and intention arise the power and capacity to really see into the hearts of others and discover the innocence of the child."[90]

I have discovered that the beginnings of anything that anyone has ever come to me about can be traced back to before the age of seven.

Your innocence as a child bought that mistaken belief, mainly because up until the age of seven—latest ten—your logical, analytical reasoning mind hadn't developed yet. You were a little feeling being only. You assumed, jumped to conclusions, and accepted whatever your caregivers believed. You didn't know any better.

You begin with surrendering and letting go of childhood resentments.

When I say that most of your beliefs and values were picked up or downloaded from your caregivers before the age of seven, there is no blame.

My mother, whose mind was not very open, used to get upset and say everybody's always blaming the parents. I would say to her, "I am not. It's just how life goes; you raise your children based on how you were raised, and your parents raised you on how they were raised and so on."

We don't go to a school to learn how to raise children. Everybody is just doing the best they can with the skills and resources they have available.

You will learn a lot in our first sessions in regards to what I call *The School Life* - your experience on this earth. The basic nature of the universe factors into how you program your mind and how behavioural change really happens.

Like how fear and your built-up emotions and limiting beliefs are running your show.

If you're a woman you may have issues with your mother—not a very good relationship or none at all (a block). So somewhere along the line you've made a decision (even unconsciously—out of your awareness) that you don't want to be a mother like your mother. Or, you decide, "I'm never going to have children." Or you are looking to have a baby to fix your relationship, make you happy, make you feel special about yourself, make someone love you, fill a missing something in your life, get you out of a job you don't like, fill a cultural expectation, or fulfill an obligation.

Maybe your partner wants to have a baby, but inside you are unsure or doubtful. Or maybe you've given up on a goal or dream of yours, and so you're not 100 percent committed, which influences the outcome.

Speaking of incongruence, often part of you wants to have a baby and another part of you doesn't. When you feel divided about an issue, it's as if you're fighting with yourself on the inside and no one part ever wins!

True happiness comes from how you feel inside and if you're looking for someone or something else to fill you up, that's when you know you're out of balance.

Do you feel *stress* is a contributing factor to your not being pregnant yet? When we talk about stress, we are really talking about your experience of what is stressful. When we consider your body as part of a stress response, it means that your body is only responding to what is held in your mind— your expectations, your way of being with life, and how you perceive your life.

The best approach to stress is to prevent it in the first place by understanding how and where it arises—which is within yourself.

It does not exist in your friend who's late, your husband of twenty years who doesn't remember what you like on your hamburger, or your mate who's not a great conversationalist. Nor does it exist in your experience of looking for a clinic to make you pregnant, or being in a bank lineup that's too slow.

As David Hawkins says, "*Stress* comes from our giving externals power over our life, which comes from the position of victim, of putting the source of our happiness outside our life and denying our power of our own mind."[91]

Having no personal boundaries, and not knowing where you need them, is a big stress factor. You need them anywhere you're experiencing drama! Like people yelling, fighting, and arguing. Or you silently fuming as you continue to listen to— over and over again—negative stories, gossip, etc.

Each time you create a clear, realistic boundary you

- claim more positive control over your time,
- respect yourself,
- increase your self-esteem and sense of personal power,
- clarify your relationships with others, allowing people in your life on your terms, and
- align your time choices with your values.

The better you understand boundaries, the more you can put them to work for you.

Each time you set a boundary, you define what you will or will not do, and you assert what you will or will not tolerate in terms of demands upon you. You're developing a limit. This is how you "make" time for what matters most and reduce stress exponentially.

There are *three requisites for permanent change*. First, you must clean up your past by disconnecting the excessive strings of negative emotions (it's the energy of your emotions and your old patterns of thoughts, limiting beliefs, and attitudes, that keep you focusing backwards) in order to bring you calmness, hopefulness, and clarity so that you can decide exactly what you want. Then, you can begin actioning—setting personal boundaries with yourself and also with others. Finally, focus, focus, focus forward on exactly what you want.

When you are in "problem" mode, you are in a state of overwhelm. Once we've handled the energy of your emotions by letting go and releasing your old anger, sadness, fear, hurt, or guilt (which in turn gives a different meaning to your past events, allowing the solution to come forward easily), your emotions will no longer be distracting.

So it's not really the event that happened that is the problem, it's the way you *feel* about it. Change how you feel about it and it changes the way you see it.

When you see for yourself through the process that you really do have control over your feelings, that you can set boundaries, and that your mind is really powerful (and by using it you can release unbalanced emotions and limiting decisions from your past), you can make profound mental and emotional changes today that will impact your future.

Releasing your emotions of guilt, apathy, grief, fear, desire, anger, and pride (to name a few), which all come from feelings of lack in your world, allows you to become freer. You will also feel *neutral* because once you are unattached to these negative, lifetime emotions and beliefs you will regain clarity and choice so that you can make good decisions again for your highest good.

Through the coaching process you

- decide to be *willing* to take a good, hard, deep look at yourself, accept 100 percent responsibility for your choices, and find that you can then overcome those self-imposed limitations. You accept what was, which in turn allows you to feel confident because you've had your life questions answered through the positive learnings gleaned from the process;
- *accept* the fact that you only have control over yourself and for yourself—not over how others behave. That's their responsibility. You're only responsible for how you respond to their behaviour;
- *forgive* yourself by realizing that you're only human and are doing the best you can with the resources you have at the time. You cope with life the best way you know how at any given age. It's okay, you're okay. Then and only then can you forgive others. Remember, it all starts with you;
- come to learn and have different perspectives and a greater *understanding* of the reasons that things happen. No, you're not being punished; all of life's experiences are teaching you.

Then you'll begin to view and experience your world as a loving, kind place. It begins to feel friendlier. Now there is the beginning of happiness and feeling good about yourself again. Self-care comes out of these changes as you take responsibility for, start looking after, nurture, and truly love yourself—no longer with blame and self-criticism.

You came here to remember who you are—an infinite, divine being in a human body, having a life experience.

Body, Mind, Spirit: A Holistic Approach to Healing

I believe true healing includes physical, emotional, mental and spiritual aspects—all of you.

I believe the world is opening up more and more to explore this concept and I am so pleased about that.

The scientific community has now shifted to a more serious investigation of alternative healing approaches. Won't it be great one day when they both work together assisting people with their whole health. Look at pharmacies—almost every one carries its own line or a reputable line of natural medicines. Meditation, yoga, massage, and new approaches to nutrition are becoming more and more mainstream in healing. And, as more and more people take responsibility for their lives and their health, the quicker these approaches will come together.

Nearly thirty years ago, Deepak Chopra said, "I see the trend toward increasing self-awareness and empowerment as a sign of expanding and collective health."[92] And he was right. Look how far we have come.

I believe that you can have a better life than what you've had so far by making good decisions.

I believe that when you make better choices, you make the world a better place for your children and your children's children.

And, I believe that with greater understanding of how life works, you'll begin to be and feel happier because you will re-own your love of self—which is where all self-healing and miracles happen.

What if you could choose to feel, hear, think, and see things differently, in order to have your best life ever?

Modalities

Neuro-Linguistic Programming (NLP)

NLP as a coaching therapy has been applied in business for many years—most world leaders are trained in it, and it is now having an impact in health, education, and sports.

NLP allows your coach to analyze your attitudes, beliefs, thoughts, and feelings in order to find out how they are affecting your behaviour and your achievements, and then help you to correct them easily.

NLP teaches you new ways of looking at and managing how you:

- communicate with yourself and others,
- deal with conflict,
- negotiate a "win-win" situation,
- become solution-focused rather than problem-focused,
- reframe situations and get a new positive perspective,
- look for the silver linings—the learnings—in all situations, and
- access your skills and resources.

"Neuro" is what you think; "Linguistic" is what you communicate verbally and non-verbally to yourself and others, and "Programming" is how you process the communications and experiences that lead you to your beliefs and behaviours.

Time Line Therapy (TLT) ™

TLT™ is one of the most powerful, practical processes and techniques for personal change and growth. Mind-body medicine and psychoneuroimmunology (PNI) studies explain the effects of your unresolved negative emotions such as anger, sadness, fear, hurt, guilt, grief, and shame, and how they affect your physical health and can lead to the development of symptoms and illness in your body. Both unwanted negative emotions and limiting beliefs such as, "I am a failure, I am not good enough, I am unlovable," influence every area of your life.

Developed in the 1980s by Dr. Tad James, PhD, these techniques quickly and easily

- eliminate painful emotions attached to memories and events in your past,
- help you learn from those events and use those positive learnings as a resource for your future,
- provide long lasting transformations,
- change how you react,
- clear your limiting beliefs that have left you stuck in your past so that you can have what you want in your life,
- change and reduce the intensity of how you perceive and respond to stress, and
- help you cope with loss, abandonment, anxiety, miscarriages, depression, and post-traumatic stress disorder.

Hypnotherapy

Hypnotherapy is a safe, fast, and effective therapy process which produces deep relaxation, laser focus, and startlingly quick results.

Do you feel stressed and anxious about your fertility and hear yourself asking, "When will I finally get pregnant?" Have you put all of your focus there and not achieved your results yet?

Then you should know that hypnotherapy

- is an awake state of deep relaxation,
- can decrease stress and anxiety,
- can improve hormonal balance and fertility results,
- gives you 10,000 times greater awareness to focus on what you want,
- is all about following instructions,
- activates the body's natural healing mode,
- improves concentration and helps you learn faster, and
- helps you obtain your results and goals faster.

The willingness to play and imagine is all you need for hypnotherapy.

Advanced Clearing Energetics (ACE) ™

ACE™ is a set of *strategies and processes* that assists you to

- discover the original *stressful event* behind your health issue,
- clear the emotional and/or physical energy behind the event, and
- help return your body to its natural energetic flow.

ACE™ answers *why we get sick* by showing you the step-by-step process that almost every disease takes. The ACE™ system allows us to quickly find and clear the underlying stress and the trapped energetic shock from the trauma, allowing you to learn from the event—sometimes in minutes. Once your health issue is gone, your body then heals itself, something it's always known how to do.

---

[90] David R. Hawkins, Healing and Recovery (Hay House, 2015), 123.
[91] Hawkins, Healing and Recovery, 120.
[92] Deepak Chopra, Perfect Health: The Complete Mind/Body Guide (New York: Harmony Books, 1990).

Chapter 4: Counseling

Becoming a Family Again

My name is Jackie, and I'm thirty-eight years old. I was born in England, and came to Canada when I was six. My husband is Marco. He's forty-two years old, and came from Chile. We've been married for fourteen years. I'm a book editor, but I don't find a lot of satisfaction in my job. Marco is a technical support worker, and he enjoys his work. I had an abortion at twenty-two while I was at university, and a few years ago I was diagnosed with scarring on my uterus. Marco smoked marijuana throughout his twenties and thirties, and was diagnosed with having a low sperm count. I didn't approve of Marco's marijuana use, and we were shocked to learn that marijuana could significantly lower a man's sperm count.

We began trying to have a child four years ago. I've had three miscarriages (at six weeks, eleven weeks, and twenty weeks), and an ectopic pregnancy. We've undergone three failed cycles of intrauterine insemination (IUI) treatment, one failed cycle of in vitro fertilization (IVF), and have now decided not to pursue further treatment. As a result of our decision, we're facing a life without children.

Personal Histories Prior to Infertility

My family life was chaotic growing up. My parents divorced when I was young, I'm an only child, and I've had no contact with my father since he left the family. My mother lives in England, and I have a close relationship with her, but she recently had a stroke which left her physically and cognitively impaired. I feel so sad and heartbroken over her illness, especially since I can't be there with her. I have a wide network of friends, many of whom have children, and we used to get together regularly for social activities.

Marco has a large, extended family. Some of them are still in Chile, but many have moved to Canada. He is the youngest of four and his three older sisters all have children. Before our infertility, our relationship with our extended family who live here was cordial, but not close-knit. Marco also had a large circle of friends, and we regularly attended social events with them.

There was some pressure by our parents and family for us to have a child, but we took this in stride. From the experiences of our family and friends, we understood the practical challenges of raising a child and we decided to wait before having one until we were sure that being parents was appropriate for us.

We used to have a deeply intimate life together before our experience with infertility. We were emotionally very close, and connected on many levels. We felt like we'd grown up together, and we were each other's best friend. Having a child meant starting an adventure, and having someone to share our lives with. A child would be a natural extension of ourselves.

Relationship Stability

Now we feel like we're grieving our pregnancy losses, and our new reality that, despite the fertility treatments, we might never have a child together. We're able to talk about our grief because that's something that we share, but we're having trouble communicating about our other feelings. This was never a problem before, but now we sometimes find it difficult to be available to listen to each other. Sometimes I find it hard to put my feelings into words because I'm afraid of hurting Marco, and I think he feels the same. At other times, I just feel too vulnerable to discuss my feelings and fears about the future.

We have also found it difficult to maintain our normal lives since our infertility. I think we've become obsessed with infertility over the years because it takes such vast amounts of time and energy, and it leaves little time for us to have the vibrant lives that we had before. I'm afraid that we're going to end up seeing ourselves, both individually and as a couple, only in terms of our infertility and nothing else.

Complementary Coping Strategies

To cope, I spend quite a bit of time just sleeping. I also take time off from work, but I feel stressed about all the days I'm missing. I don't really talk to my friends about our situation, and my mum is too sick and far away to help.

Marco spends a lot of time watching television, and he doesn't talk very much to his friends or family about our situation either. I depend on Marco a lot to motivate me out of my despair, and I sometimes think that he pushes his own needs aside so that he can help me. Marco is the stronger one, and I think of him as my protector and my rock. I feel that I'm not returning the support and comfort that he provides to me, and I wonder if he resents it.

We've both had a crisis of faith, and our relationship with God has changed. We wonder why God has turned his back on us, and why he won't give us a child. I feel like God is punishing me for having had an abortion. I still go to synagogue occasionally, and pray for forgiveness for the abortion. Marco stopped going to church after we started to lose the babies.

Social Solidarity

Before our infertility, we considered ourselves a complete family. But when we started to try to have a child, we started to feel that our lives were lacking without one. We've lost that feeling of completeness that we had before.

We find that the infertility experience is very private, and we don't want to talk about it with our friends or family. Sometimes we feel ashamed, or embarrassed, or we just don't know what to say. We've definitely isolated and insulated ourselves, and I think this has caused more sadness for us. We see our lives in a much smaller context than we used to.

We also find that we don't have as much interest or pleasure in our individual lives and in our relationship since the infertility. I think that our singular focus on working through this challenge has made us feel blasé, bored, frustrated, and angry at different times through the process.

Balanced Identity

We both feel stigmatized in different ways because we can't have a baby. I feel that I'm different from the rest of the women who can have babies; I don't have much in common with them, and I feel ostracized from their social circles. Sometimes, I think that my life isn't really important without a child. And now that I'm ready to conceive, I feel so guilty about the abortion. Sometimes, I just can't see myself in any other role except as a mother—not as a daughter, or a professional, or a friend.

As the only son in his traditional family, Marco feels that he's expected to carry on the family name and have lots of children like the rest of his relatives.

At first, he thought that his most important role in life was to be a husband, but now he thinks it's to be a husband and a father. If he can't fulfill those roles, he thinks that his life will be pointless.

We often have trouble keeping our feelings from each other. When one of us feels sad, it influences the other one, and then that starts a continuous cycle of sadness. Sometimes I see Marco sitting there just feeling so quiet and sad, and there's nothing that I can do. We're just two miserable people in the house, and we're both lost.

Relationship Polarization

Sometimes we feel so estranged and isolated from each other that communication breaks down between us. At other times, we experience the same feelings, but we don't communicate them to each other. I get very insecure about how things will work out for us long term if we don't succeed. I'm full of anxiety about this, but I don't really express or share those feelings with Marco if I can avoid it. He isn't very open about discussing the emotional aspects either, so we don't find any good solutions and just go into our own shells.

Another effect of the communication breakdown between us is that we are losing the emotional intimacy that we once had, and this is starting to affect our sexual intimacy. Because our love-making was about baby-making for so long, we've lost the fun and joy that we used to feel when we made love.

I think now we both feel emotionally and sexually awkward, and really neglected.

We also blame ourselves for our infertility because of my abortion and uterine scarring, and Marco's marijuana use and resulting low sperm count. There's a deep sadness that I can't get rid of at all. I feel that I'm responsible for not giving Marco a baby, and I think that he sometimes withdraws from me because I can't give him what he wants.

Incongruent Coping Styles

The individual responsibility that we feel for our inability to conceive is focused inwards, and we both often view our infertility as our personal problem instead of as our shared problem. There are times, however, when it's not enough to just blame myself, so I blame Marco for his marijuana use and how stupid it was. I don't know what to do with all of my frustration, so sometimes I lash out at Marco. Obviously, this doesn't help the situation, and we just withdraw from each other.

We also have different feelings about our future because of our crisis of faith. I feel like I'm being punished by God for the abortion, but I hope that through prayer God will forgive me. This gives me some hope for my future, and I feel that I might be able to move forward with my life. On the other hand, Marco feels that his relationship with his faith and God is broken. I think he's more entrenched in his despair that I am, and I think he feels considerably less hopeful about his future.

Social Isolation

Prior to going through infertility, we regularly attended social functions with our wide circle of friends. Since our infertility, we still have some contact with our friends, but our circle has grown smaller because we often avoid couples who have children. We also feel somewhat isolated from our family because we haven't been able to discuss our infertility openly with them.

It upsets me that there's a difference in the amount of support that we receive from other people. Some of my friends ask me how I'm doing, but they rarely ask about Marco. I get attention from the people who know about our condition, but no one really acknowledges Marco's pain. They all look at him as having to be strong and look after me, which he does. I don't think that I've been there for him as much as I should have been. I think Marco feels bitter about this, and about the attention I get. It comes out sometimes in the way he talks to me, or when he withdraws into himself.

Identity Disruption

I often feel that not only am I responsible for my infertility, but my body is also defective. Three times the babies died while I was carrying them. I never knew why they died, but I just knew it was my fault. It was my body; it was me who did this terrible thing to Marco and to us. I feel a part of me died, also. As a woman, I am ashamed and embarrassed and feel useless. I don't know any more who I am, or who I am supposed to be. I wonder sometimes what we are going to do now that we can't have a child. Marco also feels this way.

When he received the infertility diagnosis of low sperm count, he felt physically defective and not like the man he used to be.

We understand each other's self-blame and low self-esteem. Marco tries to compensate for my sadness by giving me more attention, but this puts more stress and strain on our relationship. Sometimes we can't seem to nurture each other, and can't look to the future because we feel trapped in the present. Marco says that everything tilts in opposite directions in our lives. We feel like our world has stopped moving forward and nothing fits together anymore. Everything is in chaos.

Next Steps

We both recognize that we're in crisis, individually and as a couple, and that we need counseling. We hope that by talking about our feelings and our fears we will find ourselves again, reconnect with each other so that we can feel the sense of completeness that we had before our infertility, and come to terms with not having a child of our own.

The Role of Counseling in the Fertility Journey;
by Reina Zatylny, MSW

Jackie and Marco's infertility story demonstrates the eight relationship characteristics that I use to assess how well you as a couple are coping with your infertility: relationship stability, complementary coping strategies, social solidarity, balanced identity, relationship polarization, incongruent coping styles, social isolation, and identity disruption. That is why I divided their story into those sections.

In this part of the chapter, I will explain those relationship characteristics in further detail, and how you can achieve a positive outcome in spite of your infertility.

When I counsel infertile couples, I address the status of eight relationship characteristics. The first four characteristics—relationship stability, complementary coping strategies, social solidarity, and balanced identities—indicate that you are able to maintain a high degree of unity in the face of your infertility.

You will very likely survive your infertility with your relationship intact, and emerge stronger afterwards. The remaining characteristics—relationship polarization, incongruent coping styles, social isolation, and identity disruption—indicate that you are not able to maintain a high degree of unity in the face of your infertility. You are having difficulty coping with it, and so your relationship might be at risk.

Relationship Stability

Relationship stability is the basis for confronting and working through the many challenges of infertility, such as making decisions concerning fertility treatments, deciding how to deal with your own fears, and determining how to get on with your lives while you are trying to have a child. It is important to understand whether your relationship was secure before you experienced infertility, and whether the two of you continue to work on ensuring stability in the relationship during infertility.

You can maintain relationship stability as a couple by making a conscious decision to be *united against a common enemy* (the enemy being infertility), creating a comfortable and nurturing atmosphere with *open communication, preserving normalcy* by compartmentalizing your issues surrounding infertility, and showing *empathy* by actively listening to each other.

Jackie and Marco can maintain relationship stability by taking care of their own well-being and the well-being of the relationship. Since the sadness and grief of facing infertility is a shared experience, and both of them are suffering at the same time, it is easy to feel emotionally overwhelmed. It will help if they can agree that they will take turns supporting each other so they both get the support that they need. This will help them become *united against a common enemy* (the enemy being infertility). Jackie has done this already by realizing that their grief is a shared experience, and something that they can talk about.

Open communication contributes to relationship stability when both of you can show mutual *empathy*, listen in an attentive manner, and provide a nonjudgmental atmosphere where each of you can offer and receive mutual, unconditional support. For example, using "I" statements such as, "I feel sad when you ignore me" is more effective than, "You make me feel sad." These techniques can help Jackie and Marco to communicate more effectively so that they feel emotionally safe, trusted, and openly vulnerable to one another.

Preserving normalcy in an infertile relationship often involves creating a new normal. When you are unable to conceive, you often need to discern and reflect on what is already meaningful in your life, and what you can do to enhance the meaning that you already have in your lives. For example, you can try to bring the sense of fun and play back into your lovemaking so that it is no longer about just baby-making.

Complementary Coping Strategies

Complementary coping strategies do not imply that you need to cope with infertility in the same way. Rather, your coping mechanisms need to be mutually respectful and supportive. Couples that are strongly committed and support one another tend to have stable relationships that can withstand the challenges of infertility. You can support each other by employing various *types of coping styles*, attending *counseling* either independently or together, relying on faith or some sense of spirituality that you might already have, and collaborating on *solution-focused problem solving* that concentrates on the facts of the situation instead of the rollercoaster emotions associated with infertility.

How the both of you cope with infertility and being without children can be vastly different. However, if your coping strategies are mutually respectful and supportive, this adds greatly to the success of your relationship. The *types of coping styles* that Jackie and Marco are using are not complementary. An effective strategy that they can try involves the "buddy system," which is based on the idea that only one partner can feel poorly at any one time, allowing the stronger partner to be available to support them. An equally matched buddy system works best so that your partner is not supporting you the majority of the time. One of you might talk about the other one as being the primary source of strength, or "my rock." However, when one of you depends so much on the other one for support, and is unable to provide the other one with it, relationships can suffer. Rocks crumble, and mutual support is necessary.

Some sense of spirituality or *faith* is often a crucial part of the lives of couples who cope successfully with infertility. If you are having a crisis of faith, like Jackie and Marco, and are trying to make sense of your lives and your place in the world, it might be helpful to discuss within your religious family how those family members came to terms with unanswered prayers and disappointment. If you are struggling with your legacy, and are wondering who will remember you when you are gone, you might find comfort by bringing children into your lives to nurture, either as godparents, or aunts and uncles, or through volunteering activities working with children.

Although grief, sadness, and disappointment are understandable emotions connected with infertility, you can use *solution-focused problem solving* to move beyond the day-to-day stresses of infertility. Jackie and Marco can start by remembering that they once viewed themselves as a family, and that they are united in their grief. They can build on that foundation by starting to plan for future activities that they would like to undertake to expand their lives in a meaningful way both individually and as a couple. Completing one of those activities can increase their confidence, generate momentum, and create a positive snowball effect.

Social Solidarity

When you feel that you are part of a world or environment larger than yourselves, you can see perspectives that will help you through many of the difficulties that you encounter. You can foster social solidarity, and feel connected with the outside world, by *viewing yourselves as an established family* even though you might not have a child, *turn to others* to share your stories with trusted people so that you can see your lives in a larger context, and keep the relationship vital by rekindling the interest and pleasure that you found in life before infertility.

For Jackie and Marco, experiencing infertility and being in a relationship without children has become an isolating experience. This is not a healthy situation for them or their relationship. As difficult as it might be, it is important that they try to *turn to others* to share their experiences. A trusted friend, family member, support group, or counselor can help them adjust to the concept of life without children. They can also consider developing new relationships with couples who do not have children to foster more social solidarity.

Jackie and Marco were successful in *viewing themselves as an established family* before their infertility, but have lost that feeling since their infertility. They need emotional flexibility to achieve this realization despite the disappointment of not having a child. They have to get to know each other in a new context instead of seeing each other as parents. Jackie and Marco had a sense of completeness before. They can achieve that feeling again if they rekindle the interests and feelings they had before their infertility, but in the context of an involuntarily childless couple. Nurturing themselves and each other will also help in *keeping the relationship vital*, and make the transition easier.

Balanced Identity

It is important for you to realize that infertility is something that is happening to you, and that you are more than just an infertile couple. The more successful couples find a way to integrate their condition into their identity, and do not define or label themselves solely as being infertile. You can achieve a balanced identity by *rejecting the stigma of infertility*, realizing that *you are more than just spouses* and are multi-dimensional individuals with varied interests and qualities, and by *differentiating yourselves from each other* by not sublimating each other's emotions and thoughts.

Jackie and Marco have not been successful in *rejecting the stigma of infertility* because they each feel stigmatized in their own way, and are often singularly focused on their infertility. They can start to deal with the stigma by using the techniques to foster social solidarity so they do not feel alone in a fertile world, such as keeping their relationship vital and turning to others for support. Using a buddy system to foster the more positive behaviors of each other can also help them overcome the stigma they feel, and integrate their condition into their identity. This requires constant work, and they will have to be vigilant against slipping back into old patterns of identifying themselves in such a limited fashion. Once they see themselves as more than an infertile couple, they can take a stand against the values and attitudes of those who consider them a failure because they do not have children.

Within their relationship, Jackie and Marco need to address the fact *that partners are more than just spouses* going through the difficulties of infertility. Working to keep the relationship vital can give them a healthier and more realistic concept of themselves, and will help them achieve a more balanced perspective of themselves and their relationship than they have currently.

While it is important for you to be empathetic towards one another, it is equally important for you to *differentiate yourself from your partner*. Jackie and Marco take on each other's thoughts and emotions, which can lead into a downward spiral toward melancholia and depression in the worst cases. They should work to develop some emotional distance, or emotional boundaries, in order to protect themselves and their relationship, and develop their own sense of autonomy and independence.

This can be accomplished in several ways:

- Realize that it is important not to give your partner more power than you give yourself, and to take back power over your own feelings. Each of you must take responsibility to work through your own emotions.
- Understand that being empathic is a loving gesture, but emotionally rescuing your partner in pain is not healthy or ultimately helpful.
- Spend time alone so that each of you can work on the parts of your lives that feel empty, insecure, or needy.

Relationship Polarization

Infertility can highlight differences between each of you that were already present, create new differences, and polarize your relationship. It is important to determine if there is instability in your relationship, and if you are isolated from each other. Relationship polarization manifests itself when communication breaks down leading to your *estrangement and isolation from your partner*, your *neglect* of your relationship, and your engagement in *self-blame*.

Jackie and Marco have withdrawn from each other because they are taking personal blame for their infertility and inability to conceive. By being emotionally and sexually withdrawn, you can become *estranged and isolated* from each other, and *self-blame* can lead to a complex array of other emotions in each of you which can result in the breakdown of your relationship. The self-interest that you show when you are caught up in your own needs, so that you are unable to attend to the needs of your partner, results in *neglect*, and contributes to the polarization within your relationship.

However distressed and fearful you feel, it is imperative that you communicate with your partner. Sometimes you might fear upsetting your partner by sharing your sentiments, but the expression of those sentiments can be reassuring to your partner who might feel the same way. If you routinely "check in" with each other to "see how we're doing," it can help reduce the neglect, estrangement, and isolation. Counseling can help you to start to re-establish your commitment to each other and to the relationship, express your needs in a healthy and succinct manner, and develop greater emotional, spiritual, and sexual intimacy.

If you have become polarized, you can also look at taking a vacation from infertility treatments or your continuous focus on your condition. It is important for you to give yourselves permission to compartmentalize your "dark" emotions, even for a short time, because doing so might help give you greater perspective on your lives. If you can agree to engage in an enjoyable or meaningful activity (including socializing) with the promise that you will revisit the situation (and the dark emotions) at a later time, you will be able to replenish your physical and mental energy, and develop more relationship intimacy.

Incongruent Coping Styles

When you and your partner are at odds in the way that you handle your infertility, you can become angry and antagonistic toward each other, unable to progress positively and work through the infertility, and trapped in your discord. The lack of harmony in your relationship is evident when you resort to blame (both directly through accusation and indirectly through physical or emotional withdrawal), are both *unable to reach out* for individual or marital counseling, and show *marked differences in hop*efulness, especially when one of you remains generally emotion-focused and pessimistic, while the other one is more solution-focused and optimistic.

Although Jackie blames Marco for his marijuana use, counseling can help her realize that, in the final analysis, it does not really matter whose fault it is that they cannot have a child. It is too late to change what they did in the past, and the real issue is how to cope with the situation today.

To avoid the unhelpful and destructive quality of blame, you can do several things:

- Reassure each other that you are both in the relationship together, and that you need to face the situation as a team.
- Remember why you love and appreciate each other.
- Discuss your frustration and upset in as neutral a way as possible.
- Realize that the decisions that each of you made in the past may have seemed necessary (such as being pregnant and having an abortion at a young and immature age) or uneducated (such as using a drug that has

long-term effects on the body), and show understanding for those decisions.

To deal with their despondency about the future, Jackie and Marco might find it helpful to talk to religious clergy about their crisis of faith. Jackie might find the forgiveness that she seeks for her past actions, and Marco might be able to reconcile his feelings of despair with the faith that he's lost.

If you are a religious couple, talking to other religious family members to understand how they dealt with disappointment and unfulfilled dreams might also provide you with guidance and solace.

Social Isolation

You and your partner can become socially isolated and retreat into your private world if you have a history of *detachment from pre-infertility external relationships*, you are constantly reminded by other families with children of *being infertile in a fertile world*, or if you have *inequality of support* where one of you receives more compassion and attention than the other one. Without the benefit of a strong support system, or when relationships with family and friends become distant, you can turn inwards and increase the risk of conflict between each other and within yourselves.

Although Jackie and Marco do not have a history of *detachment from pre-infertility external relationships*, they have retreated from some of their relationships with their friends, especially from those with children. Marco is also experiencing emotional distress because of the *inequality of support* that he receives. He finds that Jackie gets more attention than he does, and this contributes to his feelings of being alone, forgotten, and isolated.

Jackie and Marco also feel different from their friends and family members who have children, and it is often painful and wearisome *being infertile in a fertile world*. In a society where there are constant reminders of pregnancy, children, and families, being on the outside and feeling different causes them to withdraw from their society, and this creates more individual and relationship stress.

To deal with these kinds of issues, it is important for you to expand the way you perceive yourselves in your world, especially as you grow older. Human beings are largely social beings, and if each of you can begin to expand your identity, and begin to see yourselves as more than infertile and childless, your sense of optimism and hopefulness can return. You can see this expansion of identity in couples that choose to actively participate in new social activities, engage in meaningful volunteer work, and that mentor and nurture others, including children.

You can often cope more successfully with infertility by turning to and benefiting from the empathy of a strong personal support system, or by asking your counselor about joining a support group for infertile couples. You might feel like you are the only ones dealing with infertility and unable to have children, but in a support group you can learn about others who share this challenge. By interacting with others with the same condition, you might begin to feel part of a new group and less isolated.

Sometimes society offers women more emotional support than men, and male partners like Marco can feel upset, ignored, and isolated. However, if as a woman you can be sensitive to and aware of this difference of support—and show compassion, attention, and support to your partner—you will help him feel less isolated. You can also let your family and friends know that your partner is also experiencing upset, and needs their compassion and support.

Identity Disruption

You and your partner can undergo breakdowns in your identity during a period of infertility, and become disconnected from who you are. This breakdown challenges you individually, and can lead to problems in your relationship. Identity disruption can happen when you start *feeling defective* after an infertility diagnosis, when you remain *together but apart* by withdrawing to separates spaces within the relationship, or when you *try to regain control* of the situation by withdrawing emotionally or physically. If you're a man, you may resort to reckless or inappropriate behaviors to prove your masculinity, and these behaviors often polarize your relationship.

Jackie and Marco were *feeling defective* so they started to feel differently about themselves physically and emotionally. They felt hopeless about detaching themselves from being deemed infertile and unable to conceive because they took personal responsibility for their situation. This self-blame made them devalue themselves. They also found it difficult to nurture each other, and often retreated to separate spaces within their relationship which made them feel *together but apart*. By withdrawing emotionally, they were *trying to regain control* of the situation, but the end result was a polarized relationship.

When that happens, the security and well-being of your relationship can become severely threatened. You can seek the assistance of an empathetic counselor to help guide you to formulate your new identity, both individually and as a couple, and to alleviate your fear of wondering, "Who am I?" and "What are we going to do now?" Counseling can also help you to focus on "what is and what can be," rather than on "what should or could have been." You might be encouraged to focus on short-term and long-term goals that do not revolve around having children, to imagine those plans becoming a reality, and to be happy in those plans.

To regain control over your lives and feel whole instead of defective, you can begin to understand what you most value about yourselves and each other. Asking your partner what attracted them to you, can be a good starting point. Reconfirming those positive qualities can remind you of how you once saw each other, and improve how you see each other now. You can then start to redefine your lives to incorporate the experience of life without children.

Summary

If you and your partner can maintain a high degree of unity in the face of your infertility, you stand a good chance of dealing successfully with it. Having balanced and secure communication with each other enables you to confront and work through the many challenges of infertility. Being supportive and strongly committed to each other will help you create a stable relationship that can withstand the challenges of infertility. When you feel that you are part of a world or environment larger than yourselves, you see perspectives that will help you through many of the difficulties that you encounter. And you do not need to define yourselves solely by your infertility if you can integrate it into your identity.

If you cannot maintain a high degree of unity in the face of your infertility, you will often have difficulty coping with it, and these difficulties may put your relationship at risk. If there was some lack of stability in your relationship before you experienced infertility, the infertility can magnify the differences between you and your partner, create new differences, and polarize your relationship. When you are at odds in the way you handle your infertility, you can become angry and antagonistic toward each other, be unable to progress positively and work through your infertility, and become trapped in your discord. Without the benefit of a strong support system, you can become detached from your social world and turn inwards. And you can sometimes become disconnected from who you are during infertility. This breakdown challenges you individually, and can lead to problems in your relationship.

Jackie and Marco display only a moderate degree of unity in their relationship. The stability of their relationship is being helped by the way they share their grief, but they can do more to establish open communication between themselves in an empathetic environment, and they can work toward regaining some normalcy in their relationship so they are not unduly focused on their infertility.

The coping strategies that they are employing are not complementary because they are not providing the mutual support that each requires, and their crisis of faith has left them struggling to find their place in the world and the purpose in their lives. It is helpful that they once viewed themselves as an established family, even without a child, but they have withdrawn socially from some of their friends, and this is leading toward social isolation. It is important that they counteract this tendency to withdraw, make every effort to remain connected with their social circle, and consider establishing new connections with other couples who don't have children. Reaffirming the positive qualities that they see in each other, and why they were attracted to each other in the first place, can help them regain the completeness they once felt as a couple.

Jackie and Marco's identities are threatened because they keenly feel the stigma of their infertility, they have lost sight of the other aspects of their personalities in their quest for a child, and they tend to sublimate each other's feelings. They have also become emotionally and sexually withdrawn, they blame themselves for their inability to have a child, and they feel defective as human beings. At this point, they need to work to develop a more balanced view of their identities.

Even though having a child had become an important part of their relationship and identities, Jackie and Marco can start to formulate an identity without children now that they have decided to seek counseling. They can do this individually at first to reacquaint themselves with their personal interests and desires, and take responsibility for their own emotions. They can then work as a couple to nurture what they value most about their relationship so they can be a family once again.

Chapter 5: Medical Route to Conception

It Isn't Always When We Want Things to Happen; by Hoda Abu-Zeid

We had the love, we had the marriage, but we had trouble getting a baby in the baby carriage. When my husband and I married, like many couples, we talked about when we would want to introduce the next generation. We talked, we planned, and we imaginatively plotted on a personal timeline. He was adamant about waiting at least two years but I, at the age of twenty-nine, and he, at the age of thirty-four, didn't think much of it. In fact, the idea of getting pregnant somewhat petrified me—the physical and emotional changes of pregnancy, the excruciating pain of delivery, and the overwhelming responsibility of parenting. Two years of waiting seemed very palatable.

We spent those years enjoying each other—taking trips, biking and hiking during the summer, skiing during the winter, and sleeping in on weekends whenever we pleased.

After two years, it was time to live up to our timelines and at the ages of thirty-one and thirty-six, we started trying. Not being advocates of medications, especially hormone medications, we didn't use medical birth control those first two years. We relied on natural means. I also believed that avoiding such medications would make it easier to get pregnant once we actually started trying, as my body would not have to re-adjust to its natural hormone levels. After several months, however, we had no success and suddenly we were faced with an unexpected obstacle; I developed an issue that I never encountered before—bleeding between periods. Something was not right. A piercing question kept nagging at me, "Why now? Why *now* as we *just* started trying?"

This issue carried on for several months until I was finally able to get an appointment with a renowned gynecologist whom my mother knew at the hospital where she worked. Several examinations, tests, and scans revealed that an endometrial polyp was causing the abnormal bleeding, but no action was taken to resolve it. Instead, I was asked repeatedly to go in for follow-up examinations, as if there were some hope of this polyp disappearing on its own.

We had been trying with no success for close to one year past our personal two-year timeline, so we decided to see a fertility specialist. It would be at least another six-month wait, but I felt it was senseless to continue seeing the original gynecologist since no approach had been taken to resolve the bleeding. A year-and-a-half past our original timeline, we finally had a firm date to meet with a fertility physician to have her handle both the bleeding and the desire to get pregnant.

"The things we want most in life do not come without some effort"

Walking into the fertility clinic for the first time was very intimidating. I'll never forget the sight of anxious patients, some waiting to have invasive procedures and some even walking out of the clinic sobbing. In that moment, I realized that this journey was not going to be easy, either physically or emotionally.

After the polyp was removed through hysteroscopic surgery it was time to chase that elusive pregnancy, but I didn't realize how intense the journey would be. It took every ounce of energy for me to stay focused. For my husband it became intense at some crucial points, but even he was not fully aware of the toll it took on me. Cycle monitoring was quite demanding and entailed early-morning visits to the clinic for ultrasounds and blood tests. Once I understood that its purpose was to help us know the perfect time for conception, that part of the journey was more acceptable—regardless of how arduous it was. Blood test after blood test and ultrasound after ultrasound, I had to find the strength to keep going. Juggling this with work and, of course, timed intercourse was not an easy task. The mere thought of having to time intercourse was in itself stressful, as it had turned into a chore rather than an act of pleasure.

One thing I struggled with from the beginning of this journey was the fact that I would need the help of fertility medications to achieve our goal. I am not a fan of taking even the most basic of medications, especially anything that interferes with my natural hormone balance. Using fertility medications was a roadblock I had to break through.

Three consecutive months of timed intercourse with the help of an oral fertility drug was unsuccessful. With the beginning of each cycle came hope, but with the end of each cycle came anxiety. The highest peak of anxiety came each time I received a phone call from the clinic with the results of the pregnancy test. After three consecutive negative results, disappointment and frustration surfaced. However, I knew that I had to keep these emotions at bay to be successful. I also believed that some of the most important things to us in life come with some effort.

After regrouping with our physician, we decided it was time to try insemination. In some ways this gave me more hope, but in others it added more stress because I worried about my husband being available and in the right frame of mind to provide a semen sample at the clinic. At that time, he was between contract jobs and highly stressed. I knew that this would likely be reflected in the sample he gave and we were not successful in that cycle. The second cycle with insemination also failed because I only produced one follicle with the oral drug.

By the time the sixth cycle came along, things were looking up; I was given an injectable drug to try and my husband was settling into a new job, which took some of the stress off both of us. Then, to my surprise, the starting dose of that new drug led to hyperactivity in my ovaries, resulting in so many eggs that they couldn't be counted. It would be irresponsible to proceed with insemination because the chance of a high-risk multiple pregnancy (more than just twins) was very high. There was talk of converting this cycle to IVF, but it was determined that there would not be enough time to carry this through. Cycle six was wasted and we were back in line waiting for the next round.

The next cycle, my physician decided to put me on half the original dose of the drug. I somehow felt that this would be it—insemination with just the right type and dose of the drug. After all, the drug was definitely working. Also, it was cycle number seven, and seven was a lucky number.

Lucky seven lived up to its reputation. Words cannot describe how elated I was when I received that phone call from the clinic informing me of a positive pregnancy test. I remember the exact moment. I was home from work and not feeling very well as I was coming down with a cold. I was lying in bed, feeling very "un-pregnant" because I had all the symptoms of another menstrual cycle coming on—the cramps, the bloating, and the emotional changes. So when the voice at the other end of the phone said that I was pregnant, I was nicely surprised.

As soon as that call ended, I phoned my husband. He was equally excited and although we were not ready to make this public, we agreed to share the news with our parents as they knew of our struggles to reach this point. As I lay in bed that afternoon reminiscing on the journey thus far, one thought kept replaying in my head—there is nothing sweeter in life than finally achieving a goal through plenty of blood, sweat, and tears.

"Hang onto hope"

Getting pregnant was one hurdle but *staying* pregnant was another—especially after going through fertility treatment. I started bleeding about halfway through my pregnancy. Feelings of anxiety, fear, and even failure and grief struck me as I immediately assumed the worst. I rushed to the hospital trying to remember the principle I believed in—if it's meant to be, it will be. After examining me and running some tests, the emergency room doctor said, "You're threatening to lose the baby." "Threatening," I thought to myself, "this means there is still hope." I had to believe in hope. I did believe in hope. After all, hope was what kept me going throughout the entire fertility treatment.

I took the news (and hope) and followed up with my obstetrician. Ultrasounds found a strong fetal heartbeat, but I had a low placenta which was causing the bleeding. I was advised to take it easy and not overexert myself, which I vowed to do for the rest of the pregnancy.

Twenty-eight weeks into the pregnancy, however, I experienced excruciating pain in my mid-right side, near the kidney, which led me back to the emergency room. I was off work for three weeks, half of the time in a hospital bed with no real diagnosis. Doctors could not figure out what was causing pain so severe that it triggered uncontrollable vomiting. I was kept on morphine and Tylenol with codeine during this time while doctors of different specialties consulted with each other. There was talk of operating, although I wasn't quite sure for what. The only thought ringing through my head was, "What is going to happen to my baby?"

Eventually I walked out of the hospital, but throughout the remainder of the pregnancy I would experience the same pain, although not to the same extent. I was willing to put up with it because all I wanted was to get through this pregnancy with my baby strong and healthy. In the end, my wish was granted and a healthy baby boy was born.

"Stay informed—your physician is your partner"

From the start, it was very important to me to stay informed about the entire process, including understanding the reasons behind every test and procedure performed on me as well as on my husband. Equally important was to strive to understand the results and the implications. I'm inquisitive by nature, especially when it comes to the field of human health and science, so this was neither a difficult nor a burdensome task for me. It also made the journey less frustrating and kept me motivated and hopeful for a positive outcome. Doing some research and reading on my own also helped.

I learned to trust and view my physician as a partner rather than as a miracle worker. Creating life is not the work of a magic wand in the hands of a human being in a white lab coat; it is a science and the will of a higher power. Having a strong belief in this principle kept me grounded throughout the journey.

"Every challenge in life manifests with some goodness"

Failing to conceive naturally translated into a positive personal transformation within me. This I can attribute to the relationship that was built with my physician, initially as a patient and then later as a friend, and ultimately to the personal influence she had on me throughout the journey and continues to have today. Of the various people we meet, some will inevitably touch our lives. Some will stay and some will move on, but they were all meant to cross our paths for a reason.

The hurdle in conceiving occurred at a time when I was struggling with career moves, but more importantly with an inner self-conflict because I had failed to pursue my initial dream, my calling—a career in medicine. This influenced my ambition toward other aspects of my life because the fire within me was missing. Throughout every step of my pregnancy journey, I became increasingly convinced that this particular physician was placed in my path for another reason. It wasn't just so I could get pregnant; it was as if God was telling me it was time to search my soul and pursue the things in life that I was passionate about. What better way to help me do this than to place the perfect role model right under my nose; the ideal physician that I had always envisioned myself becoming.

Unlike many patient-physician relationships where time and personal connection are lacking, our relationship took a more natural course. I admired my physician for her humbleness and compassion, and the care she consistently showed to help put me at ease despite her demanding role. We connected instantly and our conversations flowed naturally, always inspiring me and leaving me with a lift in spirit.

This challenge has reinforced my belief that some of our difficulties may turn out to be good for us for reasons that may not be immediately obvious. Ironically, today I thank God that we had some trouble getting pregnant, for if it weren't for this, I would not have crossed paths with my physician and would not have become the person I am today, finally pursuing some of my long-time ambitions. This fork in the road was the game changing moment in my life.

Whatever your challenge may be, accept it with grace, pursue it with heart and soul, and always keep the faith. Look for the goodness in things, no matter how big or small and recognize that it may not be immediately obvious, but someday, somehow, it will be revealed to you.

Naturopathic Doc + Fertility Doc = Our Little Miracle;

by Tanya Wylde, ND

Our infertility story is full of heartache like many others, but we are hoping that by sharing it, you will feel less alone. We also hope that we might inspire you and give you the strength to keep trying and get the right help so that you can achieve your dreams too!

Growing up I had irregular menstrual cycles, acne and very painful periods. I also ended up in the emergency room several times with extreme abdominal pain that resulted in cold sweats and uncontrollable vomiting. At each emergency room visit, the doctors told me that I had cysts rupturing in my ovaries. They didn't say I needed to investigate further or that some underlying medical condition was the cause. They just did what emergency room doctors are supposed to do, find the cause of the emergency, deal with it and then let my family doctor address the rest.

When I was at university, my family doctor put me on the birth control pill (BCP) to help me with my hormones. She never diagnosed me with anything—she just said that the BCP would help. Well, she was right; the BCP was a wonder drug! While on it, my acne cleared up, I didn't suffer from painful periods or emergency room visits and I didn't have to worry about getting pregnant.

During my schooling, I decided to address my health with 4more natural treatments so I went to a naturopathic doctor who was able to help me regulate my menstrual cycle without the BCP. She prescribed certain herbs and changed my diet.

My periods however, were painful once again, and I had some more emergency room visits. It wasn't until I was engaged that I decided to go to my family doctor and request that he do some blood work to check my hormones. My testosterone hormone levels were apparently really high so he sent me to a gynecologist. Her solution was also the BCP, but I was planning on starting a family soon, so I didn't start it again.

After we were married, I went to a different naturopathic doctor close to our home to address my excess testosterone levels. I spent my first year of marriage, at the age of 30, taking supplements, herbs, receiving acupuncture and following a healthy diet. My acne cleared right up, and my periods were very regular and a little less painful. My naturopathic doctor diagnosed me with polycystic ovarian syndrome (PCOS) and my gynecologist diagnosed me with endometriosis. My family doctor told me that I didn't fit the typical picture of someone with PCOS because I wasn't overweight.

When I first met my husband, he was in his late thirties. He ate healthy and exercised regularly. He was extremely patient with all of my gynecological issues, including my painful periods and emergency room visits. He remained positive and never once blamed me, even though we thought it was most certainly my health conditions that were preventing us from having a baby.

After our first year of marriage, we started trying to have children because I was thirty-one years old. We had several young nephews and nieces and many of my close friends had already had children. We wanted our children to be close in age to their cousins and my friends' children. I thought for sure I would get pregnant right away since I already knew my diagnosis and had been working on my health for so long. In fact, I never once thought that I would have difficulty getting pregnant. I was raised in a family that was very active and ate very healthy. This healthy lifestyle carried into my adult life and was one of the things that my husband and I had in common.

We tried naturally for an entire twenty-four months before my naturopathic doctor strongly encouraged me to get extra help at a fertility clinic. We were too stubborn to go sooner because we thought it would happen naturally. The clinic called on day ten of my very first observation cycle to let me know that I was pregnant for the first time. The observation cycle was meant to get a baseline, by tracking my hormones with frequent blood work throughout my entire menstrual cycle (day one to day twenty-eight). At the same time, they were using regular pelvic ultrasounds to see if I was growing a healthy sized follicle and actually ovulating.

I had gone in on my day three, while bleeding, and again on day ten. I was shocked when they called me on day ten to tell me I wasn't ovulating but instead I was pregnant and my pregnancy hormones were going up. I thought this was very strange and even impossible, as I had been bleeding like a regular menstrual cycle from day one to three. Then one day as they were monitoring my pregnancy hormones, they dropped, indicating I was miscarrying. That was very disappointing but also frustrating because I didn't understand why they didn't tell me sooner that I was pregnant. But the experience gave me hope. This was my first pregnancy after two years of trying! I later figured out that it was also my first chemical pregnancy.

A chemical pregnancy is an early miscarriage when they see your blood pregnancy hormone hcg rise, but the numbers come down before you get to see your baby on an ultrasound. I went on to do another observation cycle where I was instructed to have intercourse because I was ovulating, only to find out later that we weren't pregnant. I learned that I definitely ovulate, just late, on day eighteen. This was no surprise to me. The only thing they discovered, beyond confirming that I had PCOS was that my progesterone was low. So I began using progesterone suppositories for the second half of my menstrual cycle each month when trying to conceive.

Next, I tried two medicated cycles with Letrozole. I never quite understood why they thought Letrozole would help, since from my understanding, Letrozole is helpful for women with PCOS who don't ovulate, but I apparently ovulate, just late. Unfortunately, my fertility clinic was located very far from my home and getting answers from the nurses and doctor was very difficult. Email communication wasn't an option and calling wasn't a possibility since most of the time their voicemail said they weren't accepting messages. I felt like a number and when the receptionist would call with my negative pregnancy results month after month, there wasn't a trace of empathy in her voice. After talking to a few women going through cycle monitoring at the same clinic, I learned that I was not the only one who felt this way.

When the Letrozole with intercourse cycles didn't work, the doctor recommended Puregon injections to make me ovulate more than one egg per cycle. We were told to try IUIs with these medicated cycles, where they washed my husband's sperm and inserted it via a catheter, through my cervix to my uterus when I was ovulating. On day fifteen of this new protocol of injections, I ovulated early and on my own and I became ill with the stomach flu, so they cancelled the IUI.

I was raised to avoid medications where possible and to use natural remedies to address my health whenever I could. I became a naturopathic doctor at 28 after 9 years of pre-med and naturopathic medical training. So the fact that I was even using fertility medications was hard, let alone using all of these hormone injections only to have to cancel the process. When I recovered from my stomach flu we started trying the same protocol again.

This time it was worse. While my body grew two healthy sized eggs, I bled through the cycle from day thirteen to day eighteen. The clinic gave me no answers as to why I was bleeding while my eggs were growing. I was so stressed out that I ended up dropping the liquid from one of my "trigger" injectable medications all over the floor two nights before I was supposed to have an IUI. I had to get the evening nurse to call in another prescription to a local pharmacy and then rush out to pick it up.

The morning of that IUI, I found out that my husband's sperm counts were one million compared to his previous acceptable samples. I went back for a second IUI the next day and found out his sperm counts were one million again. We discovered that there was a male factor contributing to our problem; or he was just plain stressed. I was told by the clinic that we only needed one sperm to meet my egg so his counts didn't matter. Well, I didn't get pregnant on that cycle either.

My naturopathic doctor used this information wisely and put my husband on a bunch of antioxidant supplements that he took with great compliance. After the eighth unsuccessful medicated IUI cycle with this fertility clinic we decided to take a couple of months off and then try another clinic, closer to home. Those three years of yearning for a baby we couldn't make were extremely challenging, especially when we attended social gatherings where friends and family asked when we were going to start a family. I began to isolate myself socially to avoid this question and focused more on my career, but that was also challenging because patients would ask me the same question. Early morning cycle monitoring before work became exhausting too.

When I walked into the new fertility clinic, I was so calm and relaxed that I felt as if I were walking into a spa! My new doctor had the best bedside manner compared to any doctor or specialist we had ever met. Her receptionists were available by phone during working hours and her nurses even answered my emails. They kept me informed as to my daily progress throughout my cycles and always remained very optimistic for us. My doctor had a lot of empathy for our infertility journey. She recommended that we do IVF and had a lot of confidence it would work. I was still apprehensive about IVF, so she was willing to try one more IUI cycle, this time with Clomid since we had never tried this medication before. It too was unsuccessful.

I was still afraid to do an IVF cycle. I was afraid of so many things at this point. I was afraid that after thirty-seven months of trying that we'd have one more failure, but at a huge expense. I was also worried that making a baby outside of my body would result in an unhealthy, unnatural baby. I was worried I was getting too old and that this was becoming a factor. And I was tired. Tired of cycle monitoring, tired of the monthly expenses and failures, but still not ready to give up.

My naturopathic doctor, my husband and my fertility doctor were very hopeful and gave me the confidence to follow through with an IVF cycle. My naturopathic doctor's recommendations and our healthy lifestyle changes improved my egg quality and my husband's sperm counts for months now so I figured it had to work. This was science after all! This successful IVF cycle was different from the previous injectable cycles that I had experienced. I felt extremely healthy as my hormones soared and my follicles ripened. I felt positive and confident it was going to work. My husband's sperm turned out so healthy that we didn't need to do ICSI (the procedure where they have to insert the sperm into my eggs). IVF was enough.

My fertility doctor ended up retrieving seventeen eggs from me (ten of which were mature on the ultrasound). I was in a dreamlike state during the retrieval and don't remember much about it at all, which is probably a good thing. We ended up with three healthy embryos. Two were transferred because of my older age. During the two-week wait I rested a bit, but went back to work three days after the transfer to keep my mind occupied.

Two weeks later I had an email from the nurse at the clinic, excited to report that I was pregnant!! I found out on my eight-week viability ultrasound that one of the two embryos took. I felt a small moment of grief that they both didn't take, but then I was so happy because I had never really wanted the risk of a twin pregnancy anyway. My doctor and her team were excellent at following through with any concerns I had during my first twelve weeks of pregnancy.

Now we have an amazing healthy son who makes us smile and laugh constantly. We are grateful for him every second of every day. I feel that my fertility journey has made me more patient and a better parent. I probably worry more than other parents about his health, because of my infertility and the insecurities that I developed through this process. But as he grows, I worry less. I do my best to forget about the journey and just enjoy life with our son.

If you are reading this, it's likely it hasn't been an easy journey for you either. Our advice would be to get a reputable fertility doctor and naturopathic doctor with whom you feel comfortable. Without my team, I believe we wouldn't have been successful on our first IVF attempt. Support and love each other no matter what because soon you will have a miniature version of yourself who will see that strong love you share and bond you even further.

Update from the last time we published this book:

The week that I put pen to paper and shared our "anonymous" story above and wrote my chapter "Naturopathic Perspectives" for this book was the week of Christmas 2015. That very same week we also conceived our daughter, *naturally* after multiple miscarriages! We were waiting for a frozen embryo transfer after a second IVF cycle done 2 years after our son was born.

I still feel that second IVF provided a purpose. It de-cluttered unhealthy eggs from my body; leaving one golden one (our daughter) to be plucked by my body allowing me to conceive naturally. One day we will donate the remaining frozen embryos to science or anonymously to someone desiring a frozen embryo donation. A strange dilemma but a real one that requires a chapter in and of itself.

Although our journey was kept very private; it is much easier for me to share our story now that our family is complete. I share our journey to inspire hope in others suffering from subfertility. I believe it was the power all forms of medicine and "letting go" of control that helped us to conceive our two beautiful children. It was often a lonely subfertility journey for me, because as a naturopathic doctor with a special interest in fertility and pregnancy; I was supporting other couples and families to conceive and have healthy labours. My patient's success stories inspired me but I secretly feared judgement when asked why I didn't have children yet.

My team of support included a few close friends and my health care providers. It was a very private journey for me, but in the end I found meaning in all of it. Growing up with two siblings and a single mom I learned to be self-sufficient and rarely ask for help. Through these fertility years I learned to ask for help, trust in bigger things, make amazing connections, let go of control, and find meaning in it all. I feel that surviving and thriving through subfertility helped me to learn patience in all aspects of life, process the feelings of grief more easily around slowly losing my mother to Alzheimer's and accept quarantine times through COVID19. It also motivated me to always remain up-to-date with naturopathic solutions to infertility for you and my patients. It is my wish that one day you will also be able to complete your dreams and find meaning in your journey.

If I could give a little advice; it would be to trust in whatever the universe has in store for you, that you will find meaning in all of this one day and to accept and ask for help. When you connect, ask for help, share and let go; this is when you conceive dreams and ideally babies!

The Medical Route to Conception;

by Dr. Timea Belej-Rak, BSc, Msc, MD, FRCSC, GREI

As women, we are born with all the eggs we have for the rest of our lives, unlike men, who produce new batches of sperm throughout their lives. When we have been in our mothers' wombs for about twenty weeks, we have the highest number of eggs in our ovaries—seven million. By the time we are born, we have lost the majority through "apoptosis" or programmed cell death, and we are down to one million.

By puberty we are left with 250,000 primordial follicles, or potential eggs.[93] Throughout our lifetime, we will ovulate from 350 to 480 eggs. Every month, about ten or more eggs in each ovary start growing and all of them die off, while only one, or sometimes two (that's how we get fraternal twins) grow mature enough to be released. This is in contrast to men who, unlike us, produce new sperm every three months.

While these eggs are within our ovaries, they are exposed to toxins, heat, and radiation and incur some damage to their DNA and/or internal machinery. Therefore, the ones that we release when we are older are less healthy and less likely to lead to a healthy pregnancy.[94] That is why our pregnancy rates go down as we get older, and why miscarriage rates increase with age.

Fortunately, there are things we can do to help. One is to start a family sooner, rather than later. Another is to stop harmful habits, such as smoking which can make menopause begin up to five years earlier. It also results in about half the pregnancy rates in our treatment programs. Women who smoke can also require up to double the dose of medications, so these are all really good reasons to quit now if you are a smoker. The same advice applies to men, as smoking can have a detrimental effect on sperm motility and can cause sperm DNA or chromosome damage. Taking prenatal vitamins (containing folic acid, vitamin D, coenzyme Q, and vitamin C; as well as fish oil or Omega-3), and ensuring that your iron levels are within normal limits, ensuring you are of a healthy weight, eating a balanced, healthy diet, and exercising from three to five times per week are additional things you can do to improve your fertility.[95]

In natural conception, the sperm enter the vagina during sexual intercourse, then swim through our cervix and into our uterus at around the time of our ovulation (release of the egg). The mucus within our cervix changes and becomes sperm-friendly around the time of the month that the egg is released. The sperm then swim from the uterus into the Fallopian tubes, where one sperm (out of many millions) will encounter the egg and, if all conditions are favorable, fertilize it.

The window of fertilization within the tube is about twenty-four hours but the sperm can survive in the woman's reproductive tract for up to three days. The highest chances of natural pregnancy occur when couples have intercourse during the two to three days leading up to ovulation, and diminish thereafter. The fertilized egg is now called an embryo (I love this word!). This embryo (truly a miracle of nature) moves along the Fallopian tube for about four days and arrives in our uterus on about the fifth day. Now called a blastocyst, it implants by burrowing into the uterine lining, or endometrium.

A small gland in our brain called the pituitary, releases follicle stimulating hormone (FSH) and luteinizing hormone (LH). The FSH causes one of the potential eggs to grow and develop into a mature oocyte, or egg. The cells around the developing egg in our ovary produce estrogen, which peaks just before or around ovulation. This triggers our pituitary to release LH, which causes the egg to ovulate (to be released from the ovary). The area in our ovary where the egg came from, the corpus luteum, produces progesterone, which helps to maintain a pregnancy in cycles where conception occurs. If no pregnancy occurs, the progesterone and estrogen levels fall, signaling our lining or endometrium to shed, thus producing a period or menstrual bleed.[96]

The likelihood of getting pregnant depends on thousands of factors, most importantly the woman's age. When we are in our twenties, our likelihood of getting pregnant on our own is about 20 to 25 percent per cycle. At age thirty-eight, it is about 10 percent per cycle and at forty, it is about 5 percent.

While these numbers may seem low, they still allow most of us to conceive naturally. When we need help, we are able to improve our chances over and above these numbers, or at least to the same levels, depending on which treatment we use. So focus on this and stay positive!

When a heterosexual or lesbian couple or a single woman comes to see me, we first talk about the regularity of the menstrual cycle and take a full medical history. Then we usually evaluate the ovarian reserve and a natural cycle to make sure the hormones and ovulation, as described above, are working and functioning properly. We also check to make sure the tubes are open, with a test called a sonohysterogram or hysterosalpingogram.[97] And we check for sexually transmitted diseases in the woman and in her partner, if she has one. If she has a male partner, we do a semen analysis. I now also include a nutritional assessment, as well as a functional medicine assessment[98] that addresses all aspects of health, not just the medical issues. I also offer the Whole Health Medicine Institute[99] approach, which is a more holistic and spiritual way of addressing our health, and I work with practitioners trained in naturopathy, acupuncture and traditional Chinese medicine (TCM), and mind-body therapies as well.

While I fully believe that addressing the mind, body, and spirit are all important in achieving the best outcome, I respect my patients' wishes and proceed with only conventional medical treatment if that is their preference. To that end, this chapter will focus on the medical aspects of treating your fertility concerns.

Ovulation Induction

For women who are not ovulating (usually associated with absent or irregular periods), we usually recommend pills or injections that cause ovulation, or ovulation induction.[100] One of the oldest used pills, clomiphene citrate, is an estrogen agonist (potentiator) and antagonist (blocker).[101] It makes your brain think there is a low level of estrogen so the brain releases more FSH from your pituitary gland, ideally making one of the follicles grow. Clomiphene citrate is highly effective in inducing ovulation (about 60 percent to 80 percent of the time) but the pregnancy rates are lower, perhaps due to the pill's negative, or antagonistic, properties. These include interfering with mucus production in the cervix, which makes it more hostile to the sperm and more difficult to penetrate.

There may also be negative effects on the endometrial lining, as the medication can occupy the estrogen receptors in there, although this is not very common and in my experience occurs less than 5 percent of the time. While extremely safe (it has been used since the 1960s) there are some side effects. These may include the lining effects just described, eye changes such as black spots in your vision, cyst (fluid-filled sac) formation in the ovaries, multiple pregnancy rates of about 10 percent (compared to 2 percent in the general population), mood changes, headaches, and bloating. This medication is usually taken from day three to day seven, or from day five to day nine, of a menstrual cycle. I usually suggest taking it at night to minimize the side effects, but almost all of the women I have treated with this medication over the past ten years have tolerated it without any concerns. Rest assured that you will probably be well, should you need or choose to take it.

The other oral medication recently introduced for ovulation induction is an inhibitor of an enzyme called aromatase that converts testosterone to estrogen in our ovaries. It can go by the name of letrozole[102] and is usually taken from day three to day seven of your cycle. Letrozole lowers the estrogen level, which allows your pituitary to release more FSH, consequently stimulating egg growth and maturation. It has some side effects related to the lower estrogen levels, such as hot flashes and nausea, but my patients have tolerated it very well. This medication's use in fertility is considered "off-label" because it is usually used for post-menopausal breast cancer patients, but most of the fertility clinics will have a special consent form for you to sign if you would like to use it.

Most studies show it is equally effective to clomiphene citrate, with some showing a slight superiority. Each physician will have a different preference and please feel free to discuss it with them. I have not seen a huge difference in effectiveness between the two, so it would be up to your doctor to see what they recommend. However, the final choice is always yours, as it is your body and your fertility we are enabling.

One other example of an off-label use medication for ovulation induction is an anti-diabetic pill known as metformin. Most studies show it is most helpful in women who don't ovulate and who do not respond to clomiphene citrate alone. However, it can take from six to nine months to be effective. In terms of side effects, it can be associated with bloating, nausea, gas, and diarrhea.

Another class of medications that can be used for ovulation induction is "gonadotropins."[103] These are the same hormones produced in our brain's pituitary gland—FSH and/or LH. They can be manufactured either from the urine of postmenopausal women and then highly purified, or in the laboratory using "recombinant DNA technology." This is where a cell receives a special gene (DNA) that allows it to make human FSH.

These medications are self-injected just under the skin, once a day, usually in the evening or as determined by your doctor. Sometimes twice a day may be required. It is really easy to do, just like a little prick. We usually have our nurses teach you how to do this before the start of a treatment cycle. The success rates with these medications are higher than with the pills, usually double, and the multiple pregnancy rates are also higher, about 20 percent. They are usually administered starting from day two or three of your menstrual cycle, or an assigned day one by your doctor, and taken for about eight to ten days. The most common side effects include emotional changes, ovarian cyst formation, bloating, and headache. I find that this class of medications is actually better tolerated and has fewer side effects than the clomiphene citrate pill.

While you are on these medications, we will keep a close eye on you with blood work and transvaginal ultrasounds, usually every few days or every day for a few days. This is usually done early in the mornings, before you go to work, because it can take until lunchtime for the blood work to be processed and for us to get the results. Then we can advise you of your next steps regarding your medication dosage and when to come in again. You may see your nurse or your doctor during these visits if you have any questions. Some clinics have apps that sync to your phone with the new appointment date and time, while others may have a "patient portal," so you can check your file online. This process of monitoring continues until you are instructed to have intercourse or proceed with a procedure called intrauterine insemination (IUI) or "sperm wash."

With the injectable medications, or even the pills, we often use a "trigger shot" which is meant to enhance or replace your own body's LH surge and thus trigger the egg to release or ovulate. There are currently two main formulations—a recombinant product or a highly purified urinary formulation. You would be told when to take this and then your intercourse or procedure would be timed accordingly.

Controlled Ovarian Hyperstimulation

In the previous section, we talked about how we use pills or injections to help women who do not ovulate. For women who are regularly ovulating, the pills or injections are used to produce more than the one follicle that they make on their own every month. This process is called "controlled ovarian hyperstimulation" or "superovulation." The aim is to produce more follicles, and thus increase the chances of success, by having more than one egg for the sperm to choose from. We know that not every egg that we release is a healthy egg, as evidenced by the pregnancy rates described previously, so by releasing more, our chances are increased. This also leads to a higher likelihood of multiple pregnancy, and that is why it is important to monitor your progress. We need to make sure you are not producing too many follicles, as that may put you at a higher risk of developing a higher order multiple pregnancy, like triplets or quadruplets, which are very risky for you and your babies.

Your cycle may be cancelled if you produce too many follicles, depending on which procedure you are having. This may be disappointing but it is the safest for you and your future baby. Usually for intrauterine insemination we want two to four follicles, and for in vitro fertilization (where we fertilize the eggs outside of the body in the laboratory), from six to fifteen. Sometimes, if you produce too many follicles you can also develop a condition called ovarian hyperstimulation syndrome (OHSS), where you get quite a bit of bloating and fluid in your abdomen. However, this occurs only from 1 to 5 percent of the time. The milder form is more common, mostly consisting of bloating.

Intrauterine Insemination (IUI)

This procedure, where we place the processed sperm into a woman's uterus, is referred to as intrauterine insemination (IUI) or "sperm wash." During ejaculation, the volume of the ejaculate ranges from 1.2-6.4 mL and usually includes secretions from the seminal vesicles, prostate gland, and bulbourethral glands, as well as the sperm (or spermatozoa). During vaginal sexual intercourse, the majority of this leaks out, so only the sperm enter the cervix and then swim up through the uterus and into the Fallopian tubes.

With IUI, these secretions need to be "washed" from the sperm, as they contain high levels of proteins called prostaglandins (fatty chemical compounds), which cannot be placed into the uterus.[104] If we did that, it would set off a violent cramping reaction in the uterus. We process the ejaculate to take out the sperm and put a very small amount (only about 0.3-0.4 mL) into the uterus with the best sperm. These are selected either with a "swim up" process or a "density centrifugation." The most viable or motile sperm literally swim up to the top of the tube and are then removed. With density centrifugation, the best ones are found towards the bottom. The one-to-two-minute procedure is usually painless and involves the placement of a speculum in your vagina (like we do for your PAP smear), then the passage of a very, very thin plastic catheter into your uterus, and then the placement of the sperm. Occasionally, you may experience mild cramping as the catheter goes through your cervix.

The sperm for an insemination, or even a semen analysis, is usually produced by masturbating and then collecting the ejaculate into a sterile container. This is usually done at the clinic in a private room, with appropriate visual aids. Occasionally, the sample may be produced at home. Each clinic will have its specific instructions for you.

IUI can be performed in a natural cycle for women who are using donor sperm if there is an issue with the partner's sperm (lower numbers or lower motility), or for single women or lesbian couples.

For those with unexplained infertility, or if several attempts without medications have been made, the IUI[105] is usually done in conjunction with the fertility medications (either pills or injections). They act together synergistically for those with unexplained infertility.

In Vitro Fertilization (IVF)

IVF[106] is usually reserved as our most invasive form of treatment, if all others have failed, for unexplained infertility. However, there are some physicians who believe it should be implemented sooner rather than later, as it provides us with the most answers as to why you may not be conceiving, and at the same time gives us the highest success rates. I believe it's best to use it when you need it, and when you believe you are ready for it.

In certain cases, where men have minimal sperm or where we have to retrieve the sperm from the testicles or the epididymis (on top of the testicles, where they are stored), this is our best choice. In these cases, there are too few sperm to perform IUI or even IVF. For IVF, we put the sperm in a dish with the eggs, and see if they can fertilize on their own. You need about 100,000 sperm per egg, so if there are not enough sperm for this, then another procedure, called intracytoplasmic sperm injection (ICSI)[107] needs to be performed, where a single sperm is injected into a single egg. This also needs to be done for sperm from testicles or epididimi, as those are not mature enough yet to fertilize an egg on their own.

For IVF, you will usually need to be on higher doses of the injectable medications because the aim is to produce from six to fifteen follicles. With this comes slightly more common side effects like mood changes, bloating, and the risk of OHSS. Sometimes the actual stimulation cycle may be preceded by taking the birth control pill, estrogen pills, or testosterone pills or patches; or another injection to first shut down the ovaries, before they are stimulated.

It is beyond the scope of this chapter for me to explain the intricacies of these different protocols. Suffice it to say that your physician or care provider will choose the best protocol for your particular situation. The usual stimulation starts on day two or three of your menstrual cycle and lasts, on average, about eight to ten days. At that time, you are also given the trigger shot we discussed previously. The egg retrieval usually takes place about thirty-six hours after the trigger shot and is timed accordingly. At most clinics, it is done in the morning. Usually, you do not eat or drink after midnight the previous day.

While this procedure is the most feared by most of my patients, I find that it is the most easily tolerated. The reason is that you usually get a little intravenous (IV) through which you receive pain medication and sedation for the procedure. I also give my patients a little sedative pill before they even get their IV to help them relax. I also give some additional medications before they even come into the procedure room, where I give extra local medication in the vagina in addition to the IV. I went through this procedure before we had such effective drugs and mine was not such a pleasant experience, so I want to make my patients as comfortable as I can. The procedure usually takes about five to ten minutes, and often my patients are snoring on the table, talking up a mile, or really, really happy. Many times, they don't even remember the procedure, as one of the medications is meant to help them forget.

You will have to take a day off work for the procedure due to the sedative medications, but you can go back to work or resume usual activities the next day. You also need to bring someone with you who can take you home. For heterosexual couples, the partner is usually present as he has to produce the sperm sample that will be used that day with the eggs. In some cases, we may need to use a frozen sample if we are using donor sperm, if the man is traveling and unable to attend, or if a previously frozen testicular or epididymal sample is being used.

You will usually be contacted by the clinic the next day to let you know how many of your eggs fertilized. You usually get an update on day three about your embryos as well. Fertilization rates are usually about 60 percent to 70 percent, as not all of our eggs are perfectly healthy and not all of the sperm are capable of fertilizing an egg. Also, not all of our follicles contain eggs, or the eggs they contain may not be mature. For example, if there are sixteen follicles on the ultrasound, we may retrieve fourteen eggs of which twelve may be mature, nine would fertilize, and four to five may stop dividing. So by day five, when most of us are now doing the transfers (called the blastocyst stage) we may only have about four embryos. Of these, we would transfer one to two, depending on your age; and very occasionally three in specific circumstances, such as with older patients. If there are any good ones left, then we would freeze those for future babies. We have blastocysts to freeze about 40 percent to 50 percent of the time.

Another technique that is now widely offered is PGS (pre-implantation genetic screening), where we can check the chromosomes in the blastocysts before we put them back, to make sure they are chromosomally healthy (i.e., to avoid conditions that can lead to miscarriages, or others such as Down Syndrome). Feel free to discuss this option with your doctor.

On that fifth day, or the day of your transfer, you usually arrive at the clinic with a full bladder. The transfer is usually done under ultrasound guidance and the fluid in your bladder allows the ultrasound waves to travel through to the uterus to optimize our visualization. In some clinics, you may even get to see your embryos before they are transferred into your uterus. In others, you can watch the white area on the ultrasound—this is the air and fluid surrounding your embryo(s)—as the transfer is done. It is magical! I would ideally suggest some guided meditation, hypnosis, or visualization around this time to increase the chances of success and allay any anxiety or worry you may feel.[108]

Medically, it is not totally necessary to take this day off. However, most of my patients choose to, just to help them relax. Some take two to three days and some up to the two weeks until their pregnancy test. I support my patients in their wishes to take as little, or as much time as they feel they need. (We are all different in how we experience events, and what is best for someone is not always best for everyone.)

Next comes the waiting time for the pregnancy test and the result, and I find it imperative to stay positive. I personally distracted myself from thinking about it with work and studying for my obstetrics and gynecology exam. We all have our ways of coping and your clinic has resources that you can tap into during this time.

Once you have completed your family, and if you still have more embryos that have been frozen, one of the options to consider is donating them. The practice of embryo donation is a new concept that is being further developed, and in some instances, is being treated similar to an adoption. If this is an option that you would consider, please speak to your nurse or physician, who can then provide you with more information and point you in the right direction.

Success Rates

I have not specifically stated the success rates of the different treatments, as they vary from person to person and are quite individualized. However, as a general overview, ovulation induction achieves pregnancy rates based on your age. Pregnancy rates with intrauterine insemination with pills or injections are usually in the 10 percent to 20 percent range. IVF success rates range from as little as 10 percent to as high as 70 percent depending on the woman's age and the particular factors associated with each situation.

In Closing

I hope this chapter has provided you with an overview of the medical treatment options available. There is so much more information to share, and you can find some reliable websites[109] that I have referenced for you. This cannot, nor is it meant to, replace a meeting with your doctor or specialist, who will be the best to advise you on your options and next steps. Furthermore, new information and options are continuing to emerge. Wishing you all the best on this magical journey!

Namaste!

---

[93] R. Gosden and B. Lee, "Portrait of an Oocyte: Our Obscure Origin," *Journal of Clinical Investigation* 120, no. 4 (April 1, 2010): 973-983; T.E. Vaskivuo and J.S. Tapanainen, "Apoptosis in the Human Ovary," *Reproductive BioMedicine Online* 6, no. 1 (Jan-Feb 2003): 23-35.

[94] K.T. Jones, "Meiosis in Oocytes: Predisposition to Aneuploidy and its Increased Incidence with Age," *Human Reproduction Update* 14, no.2 (Mar-Apr 2008): 143-158.

[95] Darja Wagner, "How to Improve Egg Quality" (PhD thesis, 2015); J.E. Chavarro et al., *The Fertility Diet* (McGraw Hill, 2008).

[96] I.E. Messinis, C.I. Messini, and K. Dafopoulos, "Novel Aspects of the Endocrinology of the Menstrual Cycle," *Reproductive BioMedicine Online* 28, no. 6 (June 2014): 714-22.

[97] ReproductiveFacts.org,"Diagnostic Testing for Female Infertility," accessed December 30, 2015, http://www.reproductivefacts.org/uploadedFiles/ASRM_Content/Resources/Patient_Resources/Fact_Sheets_and_Info_Booklets/InfertilityInWomen.pdf.

[98] The Institute for Functional Medicine, http://www.functionalmedicine.org.

[99] Whole Heath Medicine Institute, http://mindovermedicinebook.com/.

[100] S. Tannus, Y.Z. Burke, and S. Kol, "Treatment Strategies for the Infertile Polycystic Ovary Syndrome Patient," *Women's Health* (London: December 2, 2015) doi:10.2217/whe.15.40.

[101] Practice Committee of the American Society for Reproductive Medicine, "Use of Clomiphene Citrate in Infertile Women: A Committee Opinion," *Fertility and Sterility* 100, no. 2 (August 2013): 341-348.

[102] S. Franik et al., "Aromatase Inhibitors for Subfertile Women with Polycystic Ovary Syndrome," *Cochrane Database of Systematic Reviews* February 24, 2014.

[103] N.S. Weiss et al., "Gonadotropins for Ovulation Induction in Women with Polycystic Ovarian Syndrome," *Cochrane Database of Systematic Reviews*, September 9, 2015.

[104] R.R. Henkel and W. B. Schill, "Sperm Preparation for ART," *Reproductive Biology and Endocrinology* 1. no. 108 (November 14, 2003).

[105] ReproductiveFacts.org, "Intrauterine Insemination (IUI)," accessed December 30, 2015, http://www.reproductivefacts.org/FACTSHEET_Intrauterine_Insemination_IUI/.

[106] J.M. Goldberg, T. Falcone, and M. Attaran, "In Vitro Fertilization Update," *Cleveland Clinic Journal of Medicine* 74, no. 5 (May 2007):329-338

[107] ReproductiveFacts.org, "What is Intracytoplasmic Sperm Injection (ICSI)," accessed December 30, 2015 http://www.reproductivefacts.org/FACTSHEET_What_is_intracytoplasmic_sperm_injection_ICSI/.

[108] ReproductiveFacts.org, "In Vitro Fertilization (IVF): What are the Risks?" accessed December 30, 2015 http://www.reproductivefacts.org/uploadedFiles/ASRM_Content/Resources/Patient_Resources/Fact_Sheets_and_Info_Booklets/risksofivf.pdf.

[109] ReproductiveFacts.org, www.reproductivefacts.org, Canadian Fertility and Andrology Society http://www.cfas.ca, European Society of Human Reproduction and Embryology www.eshre.eu, Society for Assisted Reproductive Technology www.sart.org, Infertility Awareness Association of Canada www.iaac.ca, and Resolve: The National Infertility Association www.resolve.org.

Chapter 6: Donor Sperm

Our Journey to Meet Our Son;
by Melissa Blachinsky and Amanda Knegje

Our names are Amanda and Melissa, and we had our beautiful son Hendriks on April 20, 2014. This was made possible, along with a successful in vitro fertilization (IVF), because we were under the care of a doctor for fertility treatment.

Our journey to meeting our son Hendriks began in November of 2012, when we had our first appointment with our fertility doctor. We are a same-sex couple who at the time were both thirty-three years old. The reason we made that initial appointment was to consider our options in getting pregnant, and to gain knowledge of the risks in being successful, as we got older.

Our doctor was supportive right from the beginning, providing detailed information on our fertility options, age considerations, and sperm donor information, which was integral to our journey as a gay couple. We disclosed at this first appointment that we wanted Melissa to carry our baby; however, we wanted the embryo to be fertilized with my egg and donor sperm, as this reflected our vision to have our baby created by us both. Our doctor informed us that this would require us to undergo IVF, and she told us the details of the procedures and the cost associated. She also let us know that a schedule and a fertility plan would need to be confirmed once we decided we wanted to commit to getting pregnant. We left armed with lots of information to consider and many options to decide on, which was very helpful as we took time to decide as a couple when and if we wanted to get pregnant.

In the spring of 2013, we formally decided that we wanted to get pregnant, so we made a follow-up appointment with our doctor in May. We never considered another option because we had felt an immediate connection and trust with her and her clinic. When considering and selecting fertility support and assistance, professionalism, respect, and trust are pinnacle concerns because treatments are invasive and can leave an individual or couple feeling vulnerable, potentially anxious, and exposed.

At this second appointment, we formalized the fact that we wanted to move forward with our plan and with IVF. With the support and leadership of our doctor, we then worked through the details of what would be required to stimulate my follicle and egg development in myself, followed by the egg retrieval and subsequent fertilization with the donor sperm. In addition, Melissa would also be required to receive hormone support to ensure her body was ready for transfer when the embryos were ready. Our doctor prepared a workback schedule with us and made sure we were aware of every detail of the plan and its requirements. Both of us needed to take the birth control pill to prime our bodies to be in synchronization, starting in July of 2013, which would support the progression toward embryo transfer to Melissa in August. We were ecstatic that we would be able to begin our journey so swiftly after meeting with our doctor the second time, and felt that she mirrored and supported our vision.

We were also informed that due to the utilization of a sperm donor, we would be required by provincial legislation to make an appointment with a counselor to support the journey. Our doctor recommended a specialized counselor to us, with whom we were very pleased. The counselor provided detailed information on the sperm donor selection process, much of which was unfamiliar to us. We learned of the different sperm banks available, the information donors provided, and the legalities that prevailed with respect to the details of each donor. We felt that the counseling was very supportive. It assisted us in the sperm donor selection process by highlighting how important it is for a donor recipient individual or couple to articulate their major selection criteria. Selecting a donor can be a stressful fertility choice, as this is a major component in the physical attributes that your child may have.

After the counseling session, we felt we were more prepared to make a selection and had determined what was important to us in our choice. Melissa's family is Jewish and of Israeli descent, therefore it was important to us that our donor be Jewish, and have similar physical attributes to her family, since the sperm would be combined with my egg. We made the sperm donor selection an enjoyable and fun experience by remembering that physical and health attributes are but one component of the creation of a healthy child. Our love and family would be more significant than anything else. We made our selection based on the criteria we had established, and on a very touching letter written by our donor that was very supportive of families who required donor support to make a baby.

Once the donor selection had been made and our reproductive cycles had been synchronized, we progressed to the IVF process. In order to prime me for follicle/egg production, I was required to inject daily fertility medication (hormones) via needle in the abdomen, as well as make daily, early morning visits to the clinic for follicle development monitoring through internal ultrasounds. The level of fertility medication required by injection on a day-to-day basis was quantified and measured against the number and size of the follicles that were identified every day by an ultrasound technician, and reviewed by our doctor. The early morning appointments were difficult and anxiety-provoking because we were nervous about realizing success and progression. The clinic staff and surroundings were calming, reassuring, and peaceful, which mitigated our stress and feelings of being vulnerable. This was especially beneficial for me, as I was solo for most morning appointments because Melissa could not always accompany me due to early morning work commitments.

The impact of my being on the pill to synchronize both Melissa's and my cycle was that follicle production was slow to progress, which put this initial cycle at risk. Hearing this feedback in the first week was highly disappointing for both of us, so the monitoring was extended beyond the first week with increased levels of fertility medication by injection. This was balanced by our doctor, otherwise it could have resulted in ovarian hyperstimulation syndrome (OHSS).

The fertility medication had a profound effect on my body and emotions, causing increased emotional sensitivity, stress, and mild abdominal bloating. However, for us the result of our fertility medications was positive and successful in our journey. The stimulating hormone assisted in the production of twenty-three follicles, which were scheduled for extraction on the fourteenth day of our cycle monitoring. I was especially relieved with this news, as the fertility medication and daily monitoring was overwhelming at times.

The egg/follicle retrieval was scheduled in the early morning, thirty-six hours after the final injection. We both arrived and met with our doctor to review everything. I was mildly sedated to undergo the procedure, which entailed the retrieval of the eggs from the ovaries utilizing a needle connected to a suction device. The procedure included moderate pain with the sensation of internal pressure during the extraction, followed by mild cramping the day after.

This day at the clinic was one of the most pleasant medical experiences we have had to undergo, due to the support and attentiveness of the staff, the information provided by our doctor, and the care during and after the procedure. We were informed that the eggs would be reviewed and those that were deemed mature would be utilized and fertilized with the donor sperm, which would result in embryos.

Our fertilization was achieved using two methods: insemination (egg and sperm mixed and incubated) and intracytoplasmic sperm injection (ICSI) whereby sperm is injected directly into a mature egg. The embryos developed over a five-day period, during which time we were given updates on their progression. After five days, we were informed that we had five mature and viable embryos, which were all rated on their quality.

We were also told which were the top two embryos, as we had the choice to transfer one or two of the embryos into Melissa. The general practice and choice with individuals undergoing fertility treatment in Ontario is to transfer two embryos. This is because most individuals who are in the process of IVF, are there because of fertility constraints or difficulty, and double transfer increases the success rate of getting pregnant.

We had come to our doctor because we were a same sex couple, and inherently required fertility assistance. This was because of the need for donor sperm and to support our vision that our baby be carried by Melissa using an embryo fertilized by my egg. Due to these preliminary considerations and the increased rate of multiple births with double-embryo transfer, our decision was to opt for single-embryo transfer.

On the sixth day after fertilization, our top-rated single embryo was transferred into Melissa utilizing a catheter, which was inserted into her uterus. It was a fairly painless procedure, although it required a full bladder to assist in viewing the uterus. Although this proved to be stressful and challenging for Melissa, it also provided much-needed comic relief for both of us on that day.

Once the transfer was complete, we were required to wait twelve days to take a blood test to confirm whether the embryo had implanted into the lining of Melissa's uterus, resulting in a successful preliminary pregnancy. We both remember those twelve days as the longest in our lives. Many couples or individuals may choose to take an independent pregnancy test, which is a personal choice, however, it can result in false positives or negatives and therefore has unhelpful emotional impacts. We decided to wait the twelve days and take the formal blood test at our doctor's office.

Melissa's blood was drawn at the clinic on the twelfth day after the transfer, and we were informed that the results might come in that afternoon or the next morning. Again, we were faced with one of the longest and most emotionally taxing days, waiting to find out if we were pregnant and our journey would progress closer to meeting our child. It was on this fateful afternoon that Melissa received a call from the head nurse from our doctor's clinic confirming that we were indeed pregnant. We were a fortunate case that had resulted in a successful pregnancy on our first IVF cycle, which sadly is not the case for many individuals, but happily the result in our journey. When we had the opportunity to speak that day, as we were both working, it was one of the most joyous and cathartic conversations, full of hope but also trepidation.

Becoming pregnant was a brilliant blessing; however, knowing the inherent risks of early pregnancy, and how much we had invested, the stress and anxiety was ever-present in both of us. Like any journey, we hit milestones toward the end result (in this case meeting our son) but we celebrated cautiously because our pregnancy was not without setbacks. Melissa had a significant bleed within six weeks of finding out we were pregnant, causing alarm and fear of miscarriage. We underwent an early ultrasound which provided the feedback that medically the pregnancy was still viable. In addition, Melissa was diagnosed with kidney stones at nineteen weeks pregnant, which presented initially as a potential risk to our pregnancy and baby. Once diagnosed, we were relieved to know our baby was healthy; however, this still resulted in significant pain for Melissa. When we hit thirty-four weeks pregnant, Melissa's blood test showed a high level of bile, which was a precursor for intrahepatic cholestasis of pregnancy. This can be very dangerous to a fetus, so our obstetrician recommended early delivery.

In the end, we met our son Hendriks at 12:41 a.m. on April 20, 2014, after Melissa had labor induction and an emergency C-section delivery. Our son was and continues to be brilliant and fully healthy. We are forever grateful for modern science, our doctor, and every clinician who played a part in our journey to creating and meeting our son.

A Patient Guide to Donor Sperm;
by Haimant Bissessar

The first reported case of successful artificial insemination with human sperm was reported in 1790 by renowned Scottish anatomist and surgeon Dr. John Hunter, who inseminated the wife of a linen draper using her husband's sperm.[110] The first reported case of a woman inseminated with donated sperm (donor insemination) was reported in the American journal Medical World in 1909, although the procedure was performed at the Jefferson Medical College in Philadelphia in 1884. The author, Addison Davis Hard, claimed that a Dr. William Panacoast inseminated the wife of a local merchant who was azoospermic (without sperm, or sterile) with sperm from the best-looking medical student at the college. It was only after the pregnancy was confirmed that the husband was told that sperm from a medical student was used for the insemination. At his request the wife was never told.[111]

The possibility of freezing sperm was first observed in 1776, when the Italian priest and physiologist Lazzaro Spallanzani observed that human sperm cooled by snow became motionless and regained motion when warmed.[112] It was not until 1866 that the idea of human sperm banks was contemplated by Italian neurologist and physiologist Dr. Paolo Montegazza, who observed that human spermatozoa survived after exposure to a temperature of -15oC. He speculated that sperm could be frozen, stored, and used at a later time—in essence the creation of sperm banks. Furthermore, he suggested that perhaps sperm from men who died in battle could be used later to impregnate their wives.[113]

The sperm freezing process was refined in the late 1940s and early 1950s by British and American scientists. In 1949 Christopher Polge, a graduate student in London, England, serendipitously discovered that if he added as little as 10 percent glycerol to a suspension of rooster sperm and then froze it to -80˚C, almost all of the sperm swam normally when thawed.[114] The freezing process was further refined in 1953 by American scientists Dr. Jerome Sherman and Dr. Raymond Bunge, who froze human sperm with 10 percent glycerol on dry ice and reported a 67 percent survival rate. They subsequently reported three pregnancies from artificial insemination using frozen and thawed sperm.[115]

It was not until the 1970s that sperm banks were established with the primary focus being to cryopreserve semen samples from men prior to sterilization procedures. Cryopreservation means preservation by freezing, storing at extremely low temperatures (-150˚C to -196˚C), and thawing.[116]

Donor Sperm Use

Therapeutic donor insemination (TDI), or donor insemination (DI), and invitro fertilization (IVF) are appropriate treatment options to achieve a pregnancy using donor sperm.[117] Couples use donor sperm in situations where the husband or partner has no sperm cells (azoospermia), very few sperm cells (oligozoospermia), significant sperm abnormalities, difficulty ejaculating, a sexually transmissible infection that cannot be treated, or a genetic problem that his children could inherit. Single women and same-sex female couples who want a biological child also use donor sperm.[118]

Semen Regulations

The identification of human immunodeficiency virus (HIV) and the subsequent acquired immunodeficiency syndrome (AIDS) epidemic among young, previously healthy homosexual men in the early 1980s,[119] provided the impetus for a review of the use of donated sperm. The practice of using fresh semen (sperm cells and fluids) samples for insemination/IVF was deemed unacceptable due to the risk of HIV transmission. To minimize the risk of transmission of infectious diseases, guidelines and regulations to address donor recruitment and semen processing were developed and universally accepted. These guiding principles protected not only the health of women using donor sperm, but also children born through its use, and society in general.[120]

The regulations are enforced by government health ministries in different countries. In the United Kingdom, enforcement falls under the mandate of the Human Fertilisation and Embryology Authority (HFEA), while in the United States, it is the Food and Drug Administration (FDA) in accordance with Title 21 Code of Federal Regulations (CFR) Part 1271.[121] In Canada, the authority rests with Health Canada (HC) in accordance with regulations including the Safety of sperm and ova regulations (2019)[122] and the Assisted Human Reproduction Act (2004).[123] In Australia, enforcement is at a state or territory level, although the Australian federal government, through the National Health and Medical Research Council (NHMRC), issued national Ethical Guidelines on the Use of Assisted Reproductive Technology in Clinical Practice and Research in 2004, with revisions in 2007.[124]

Who are the Donors?

Sperm donors are typically healthy men under the age of forty-five, in good health and a low risk of genetic disease transmission. In Canada, there is no upper age limit for sperm donors.[125] in the United Kingdom donors are between eighteen and forty-six[126], and in Australia, between eighteen and forty-five, except for Victoria state where the range is from twenty-one to forty-five years.[127] The age restriction of sperm donors to around forty-five years old is based on research that found an increased risk of attention-deficit/hyperactive disorder and autism spectrum disorder (ASD) when paternal age at conception was greater than forty-five.[128] These heightened risks attributed to increased paternal age, are likely the result of the accumulation of genetic mutations in sperm cells.[129]

The priority is to select healthy men, evaluate them based on personal and sexual history by using a structured questionnaire, and exclude men who might be at high risk for HIV, sexually transmitted diseases, or other infectious agents that can be transmitted through semen.[130] The prevalence of sexually transmitted and genetic diseases may differ in different countries, so testing requirements in one country may not be appropriate in others.[131] In some countries men who have had sex with other men, who have been excluded permanently from donating blood, or who engage in sex in exchange for money or drugs, would be prohibited from being accepted as sperm donors.[132]

The screening process requires the prospective donor to complete an extensive questionnaire that includes questions on medical health, sexual history, lifestyle, and family/genetic history going back three generations (donor, parents, and grandparents). Psychological evaluation and counseling by a qualified medical professional should be undertaken to assess any psychological risks and evaluate for any financial or emotional coercion,[133] although Canada does not require it. The donor will also be encouraged to discuss his feelings regarding disclosure of his identity and his plans for future contact with children born from his donations.

The next step in the process is for the prospective donor to provide several semen samples that will be analyzed, frozen, and thawed to assess sperm quality and survival. Sperm cells are susceptible to freezing damage, and motility after thawing is generally from 25 to 40 percent.

This is followed by interviews with sperm bank personnel, a psychological evaluation, and genetic and infectious disease screening or testing. The intent of donor testing is to prevent the transmission of infectious diseases to users and to safeguard public health.[134] Some of the infectious diseases for which testing is performed are human immunodeficiency virus (HIV) types 1 and 2; human t-lymphotropic virus (HTLV) types 1 and 2; hepatitis B and C, syphilis, Chlamydia trachomatis; Neisseria gonorrhea; culture and sensitivity; and Cytomegalovirus (CMV).[135] Genetic testing is not a regulatory requirement in some countries such as Canada and the United States,[136] although it is recommended by guidelines and/or standards developed by professional organizations such as the American Society of Reproductive Medicine (ASRM), and the American Association of Tissue Banks (AATB)[137]. Although it is not possible to test for every genetic disorder, donors recruited at most commercial sperm banks undergo testing for the most common genetic disorders as indicated by the donor's ethnic background. For example, prospective donors of Eastern European (Ashkenazi) Jewish heritage may be tested for a panel of genetic diseases which include cystic fibrosis, Canavan disease and Tay-Sachs disease.

By law, sperm for assisted conception (a reproductive technique performed on a woman for the purpose of conception, using semen from a donor who is not her spouse or sexual partner) must be frozen and quarantined for at least 180 days. The donor must test negative for infectious diseases including HIV before the semen can be released for use by the recipient.[138]

The acceptance rate of men who complete the rigorous screening and testing process and are approved as sperm donors is less than 4 percent.[139] In some cases, sperm banks have reported acceptance rates as low as one in 200 men.[140]

Selecting a Donor

Choosing a donor is a very important decision and it can be a daunting and overwhelming process. Some of the questions that you may have are:

- Is the use of donor sperm legal?
- Which sperm bank should I use?
- Is a non-identity release (anonymous) donor (unknown to the recipient and/or offspring) a better choice than an identity- release donor (identifying information is made available to individuals born from these donors)?
- Should I choose a donor who was paid for his donation versus one who was not (altruistic donor)?

- What is the pregnancy rate?
- What is the pregnancy limit per donor?
- What information is available on donors and will the sperm bank help me select a donor?
- Can I use the same donor to have another child (sibling pregnancy)?
- Are donor registries or forums available?

Legality of Donor Sperm

In most Western countries the use of donor sperm in assisted conception is not prohibited by law. A law in Italy (Law 40/2004) that had prohibited gamete (egg and sperm) donation since 2004 was reversed in April 2014, allowing patients access to donor sperm.[141] In Denmark, single and lesbian women were prohibited from being inseminated with donor sperm until the law changed in 2007.[142]

All sperm banks must be compliant with the regulatory requirements in the countries where they distribute their donor perm. In some countries, only identity-release and altruistic donors are permitted, while in other countries, donors must be anonymous and unpaid.[143] Each sperm bank will have its own policies on how they manage donor recruitment, donor information, and how client complaints are addressed. The identity of women who use donor sperm is never released to the sperm donor. An important question to ask is whether the donor is required to provide medical updates, and under what circumstances is this information released to parents of donor-conceived individuals.

Non-ID (Anonymous) or Identity-Release Donor (ID Donor)?

The choice of a Non-ID donor or an ID donor may not be an option, as regulations in some countries mandate the types of donors that are available and can be used by patients. Both Non-ID and ID donors are unknown to the recipient. However, ID donors provide identifying information which is collected and kept by the sperm bank or central registries and released to the child at age eighteen.

In the United Kingdom, all donors were required to be ID donors on April 1, 2005. The HFEA, the independent regulator overseeing the regulations, collects identifying and non-identifying information on the donors.[144] Similar regulations exist in Ireland, Sweden, Finland, The Netherlands, Germany, Switzerland,[145] and the Australian states of Victoria, New South Wales, South Australia, and Western Australia.

If ID donors are mandated by regulations, then they are required to provide identifying information such as their name, address, and date of birth, which is kept in national registries and accessible to donor-conceived individuals once they reach the age of eighteen. Non-ID donors who donated prior to the introduction of ID donor legislation can voluntarily provide information about themselves to the registries.[146] For jurisdictions where ID donors are not mandated by law, the donor may volunteer to provide identifying information for release to any children born from his donation. In this case, the responsibility of collecting and storing the information is with the sperm bank. In these situations, the term ID donor may have a different meaning depending on the sperm bank chosen.

Some banks may release the donor's contact information to the adult offspring as long as the child's birth was registered with them; however, they will not mediate contact. Other sperm banks may allow the donor to share the identifying information voluntarily and they may act as a liaison between the donor and adult offspring.[147] It is important to clarify the identity-release policy with the sperm bank of your choice.

In other countries such as France, Spain, and Greece, only anonymous donors are allowed.[148] A revision to Danish fertility law[149] in 2012 allowed for both anonymous and identity-release donations, making the Danish policy similar to that of Canada and the United States. However, in 2015, due to patients' efforts, a law was introduced in Washington state that requires donors to be identity-release unless they choose to opt out.[150]

Are Donors Paid for Their Donation?

The issue of donor compensation has inspired much debate over the past twenty years and has had a profound effect on donor recruitment. In Canada, the Assisted Human Reproduction Act, enacted by the Parliament of Canada in 2004, makes it a criminal offence to purchase or advertise for the purchase of sperm from a donor, directly or indirectly.[151]

Similar criminal provisions exist in the United Kingdom, where sperm donor reimbursement was frozen at the 1991 rate of £15 plus reasonable expenses.[152] This restricted payment legislation significantly affected donor recruitment and resulted in a reliance on imported sperm. In Canada, over 80 percent of the sperm samples distributed are imported from the United States.[153] Similar shortages of donor sperm exist in Australia with the majority of sperm being imported from the United States.[154] In the UK, the reliance on imported sperm from Denmark was categorized as the "Viking invasion."[155]

However, in April 2012 the HFEA raised compensation per donation to £35 plus additional remuneration for travel expenses due to patient advocacy and the growing problem of British citizens traveling abroad for treatment.[156] In September 2014, the creation of a national sperm bank was established to be run by the National Gamete Donation Trust (NGDT)[157], a registered charity in the UK, and the Birmingham Women's Hospital. A year later only nine donors were recruited,[158] highlighting the difficult task of recruiting sperm donors. After five years of recruiting sperm donors, The London Sperm Bank (established in 2010) was finally able to report in May 2015 that domestic patients would no longer have to rely on imported sperm from Denmark or the United States. They had sufficient stock to supply clinics registered within the HFEA.[159]

In France, donors are anonymous and altruistic (unpaid) and sperm banks are part of a public network called Centres d'étude et de conservation des oeufs et du sperme humains (CECOS), which was created in 1973.[160] The operation is based on the main principles formulated by founder Georges David: "*All sperm donations must be given voluntarily without payment and the donation must come from a couple who has had one or more children.*"[161] The 2011 revision of the bioethics law (Loi#2004-800), first enacted in 2004, maintained the principle of anonymity and non-payment to donors.[162]

Pregnancy Rates

Pregnancy rate per cycle with donor insemination is between 8 and 26 percent and is dependent on many factors. These include female fertility indicators such as tubal disease, fibroids, ovulation dysfunction or endometriosis, the woman's age at time of insemination[163], and whether intracervical or intrauterine inseminations, or one versus two inseminations, were performed in the cycle. As a woman ages, the number of eggs in the ovaries declines from about one to two million at birth to a few hundred at menopause. After age thirty-five, women are less likely to become pregnant and more likely to have a miscarriage as the egg quality decreases due to chromosomal anomalies.[164]

Pregnancy rates may be significantly higher with intrauterine insemination (IUI), where the sperm is deposited directly into the uterus and Fallopian tubes, than intracervical insemination (ICI), where sperm is deposited around the cervix and the ovaries are stimulated by medication.[165] However, in natural cycles where the ovaries are not stimulated by medication, there may be no substantial benefit to intrauterine insemination over intracervical insemination.[166]

In order to perform an intrauterine insemination, the seminal plasma must be removed from the sample. An ejaculate consists of sperm cells and seminal plasma, which are fluids secreted by the seminal vesicles and prostate. The seminal plasma contains hormone-like chemicals called prostaglandins which can cause uterine contractions. The seminal plasma can be removed from the ejaculate prior to freezing or after thawing of the frozen sample. This is most commonly accomplished by "sperm washing," whereby the sample is transferred into a test tube and spun in a centrifuge so that the sperm cells form a pellet at the bottom of the test tube. The pellet is then re-suspended in a special fluid known as the media, and drawn up in a catheter for insemination.

Home Insemination

Patients may opt to perform at-home self-insemination with donor sperm for a variety of reasons. These include the significant costs of attending a fertility clinic when there are no indications of fertility issues to prevent a pregnancy, the unavailability of medical services such as in a remote area, and the denial of fertility services to women based on sexual orientation and marital status.[167]

Some sperm banks in the United States and Canada will ship frozen sperm samples to home addresses for at-home insemination and provide an insemination kit (gloves, syringe, and catheter), instructions on how to thaw, and the insemination procedure. In most cases the sperm bank requires that the patient be under the care of a physician, and the physician must authorize the shipment of sperm.[168] Other banks, such as Cryos International in Denmark, do not require the patient to be under a physician's care.[169]

In the UK, the shipment of sperm for at-home insemination is regulated by the HFEA. Only under exceptional circumstances (the reasons must be documented in the patients' medical records) will sperm be released for at-home insemination. The sperm sample must be thawed or thawing, and cannot be shipped in any container that would preserve the sperm in a frozen or preserved state.[170]

Since women may not have the ability and equipment to "wash" the sperm, or perform an intrauterine insemination, most at-home inseminations are typically intracervical inseminations.

There has been limited research to determine if the pregnancy rate per cycle increases when two inseminations are performed on consecutive days versus a single donor sperm insemination. One of the early studies showed an increased pregnancy rate, while other studies showed no difference in pregnancy rates.[171] A recent large study (where 673 single inseminations were performed on 235 patients, and 2,486 double inseminations were performed on 896 patients) concluded that there was no statistically significant difference in clinical pregnancy rates.[172]

Pregnancy Limits

It is common practice to look at "family units" rather than children or pregnancies resulting from donor insemination. A family unit can have multiple children from the same donor and still be counted as one family unit. Some locations, such as the United Kingdom[173] and the state of Victoria in Australia[174], have a maximum of ten families from one donor. The limit in New South Wales, Australia is five family units,[175] and in France it's no more than ten children. There are no limits in Canada, Sweden, and the United States, although the 2013 American Society of Reproductive Medicine (USA) recommendations suggest that, "*It is difficult to provide a precise number of times that a given donor can be used because one must take into consideration the population base from which the donor is selected and the geographic area that may be served by a given donor. In a population of 800,000 limiting a single donor to no more than twenty-five births would avoid any significant increased risk of inadvertent consanguineous conception*" 175 (inadvertent half-sibling unions between the offspring). An international working group looked at genetic, psychosocial, operational, and ethical considerations and recommended that for a sperm donor that is used internationally, "*the offspring number created per donor should be limited to no more than one hundred families*."

Available Donor Information/Selection Assistance

The previous routine of clinical personnel or physicians selecting and matching the recipient to the donor is no longer widely practiced. Patients choose their own donors, which involves direct contact with sperm banks or the importer/distributor. In order for individuals to make an informed decision, donor information must be easily accessible. Sperm banks and donors provide detailed medical history profiles and personal profiles which contain information on donors' hobbies, family background, interests, likes, dislikes, physical characteristics, childhood and adult photographs, handwriting analysis, and audio recordings of the donor's voice.[176] The information is easily accessible on the sperm banks' websites at a nominal cost or free of charge. Assistance to select a donor is also provided by the sperm banks and importers/distributors.

Sibling Pregnancies-Can I Use the Same Donor?

There is a trend with sperm banks to reduce the number of samples that a donor can provide.[177] In part, this trend is to address the concern that a large number of babies could be born from the sperm of a single donor. Therefore, if you are contemplating having more than one child with the same donor, you may want to consider storing multiple vials of sperm at your sperm bank for future use. There is no guarantee that sperm from the donor used to conceive your first child will be available for future siblings.

Sibling Registries

Sperm banks may offer post-conception services such as forums or registries so individuals conceived through the use of donor sperm can make contact with others with whom they share genetic ties. While each sperm bank may have its own forum or registry, the most internationally recognizable and well-known registry is the Donor Sibling Registry (DSR) created in 2000 by Wendy Kramer and her donor-conceived son Ryan in Colorado. DSR is a non-profit, member organization, not affiliated with any sperm banks, whose goal is to "*advocate for the right to honesty and transparency for donor kids, and for social acceptance, legal rights and valuing the diversity of all families*."[178] At the DSR website, donors, donor-conceived people, and women who have used donor sperm can engage in discussions, post messages and ask questions.[179] A similar organization, the Donor Conception Network in the UK, also offers support to families and children conceived with donated sperm, eggs, or embryos.[180]

Conclusion

The laws, regulations and guidelines that surround the recruiting and screening of sperm donors and testing for infectious and genetic diseases varies in different countries, and in some cases within countries. In some countries, only ID (identity-release) donors are allowed while in others it's strictly non-ID (anonymous) donors, and in a few countries both anonymous and identity-release donors are allowed to donate sperm.

With increasingly stringent regulations and the prohibition of payment to donors, the trend has led to shortages of sperm samples, which has forced the importation of sperm samples from abroad. In situations where using donor sperm to build a family was illegal, individuals were forced to travel abroad to seek treatment. More recently, regulatory changes in some countries have removed barriers to treatment and reduced reliance on imported sperm.

Many of the regulatory changes have been patient-driven. In the United Kingdom, after considering the evidence provided by patients and supporters, HFEA raised the compensation offered to donors to £35 per visit.[181] In Italy, the court's decision to change Law40/2004 "*was based on the new vision of how to promote patients' interests.*"[182] In France, a 2011 review of the legislation reaffirmed that sperm donors will remain anonymous.[183] Patient input will be integral and invaluable to the shaping of future legislation.

Ultimately, the final choice in selecting a donor to build your family is yours, and your decision will be influenced by sperm bank policies, available donor information and regulations in your jurisdiction.

---

[110] Sonia Fader, "Sperm Banking: A Reproductive Resource," (1993), http://www.cryobank.com/Learning-Center/Sperm-Banking-101/Sperm-Banking-History/.
[111] Ibid.
[112] J. Barkay and H. Zuckerman, "The Role of Cryobiology in Artificial Insemination," in *Human Artificial Insemination and Semen Preservation*, eds., D. Georges and P. David (Paris: Plenum Press, 1979).
[113] C.C. Polge, A. Smith, and A. Parkes, "Revival of spermatozoa after vitrification and dehydration at low temperatures," Nature 164, (October 15, 1949): 666, doi:10.1038/164666a0.
[114] A. Pacey and M. Tomlinson, *Sperm Banking: Theory and Practice* (Cambridge Press, 2009), 4.
[115] Michael J. Tucker, "The Freezing of Human Oocytex," http://www.ivf.com/freezing.html.
[116] American Society of Reproductive Medicine, "Recommendations for gamete and embryo donation: a committee opinion," *Fertility and Sterility* 99, no.1 (January 2013): 47-62.

[117] *Third-party Reproduction: Sperm, egg, and embryo donation and surrogacy. A Guide for Patients* (Alabama: American Society of Reproductive Medicine, 2012), 9-10.
[118] J.W. Akin et al., "Initial experience with a donor egg bank," *Fertility and Sterility* 88, no. 497 (2007): el-4; National Institute of allergy and infectious diseases, "The Relationship Between the Human Immunodeficiency Virus and the Acquired Immunodeficiency Syndrome," accessed January 29, 2016, http://www.niaid.nih.gov/topics/hivaids/understanding/howhivcausesaids/pages/relationshiphivaids.aspx.
[119] Government of Canada, Justice, "An Act respecting assisted human reproduction and related research," (2004), https://laws.justice.gc.ca/en/a-13.4/2389.html; Human Fertilisation and Embryology Authority, "HFEA agree new policies to improve sperm and egg donation services," (2011), http://www.hfea.gov.uk/6700.html; Australian Government, National Health and Medical Research Council, "Ethical guidelines on the use of assisted reproductive technology in clinical practice and research," (2007), https://www.nhmrc.gov.au/_files_nhmrc/publications/attachments/e78.pdf.
[120] U.S. Food and Drug Administration, "What You Should Know - Reproductive Tissue Donation," (2010), http://www.fda.gov/BiologicsBloodVaccines/SafetyAvailability/TissueSafety/ucm232876.htm; Alyce. C. Katayama, "U.S. ART Practitioners Soon to Begin Their Forced March into a Regulated Future," *Journal of Assisted Reproduction and Genetics* 20, no. 7 (2003): 265-270.
[121] Health Canada, "Safety of sperm and ova regulations.," (2019), https://laws-lois.justice.gc.ca/eng/regulations/SOR-2019-192/index.html
[122] Government of Canada, Justice, "An Act respecting assisted human reproduction and related research,"(2004), https://laws.justice.gc.ca/en/a-13.4/2389.html.
[123] Australian Government, National Health and Medical Research Council, "Ethical guidelines on the use of assisted reproductive technology in clinical practice and research," (2007), https://www.nhmrc.gov.au/_files_nhmrc/publications/attachments/e78.pdf.
[124] American Society of Reproductive Medicine, "Recommendations for gamete and embryo donation," 48.
[125] Human Fertilisation and Embryology Authority, "HFEA agree new policies".
[126] Sperm Donor Australia, "Are You Eligible? Who Can Be a Sperm Donor," (2015), http://www.spermdonorsaustralia.com.au/who-can-donate/are-you-eligible/.
[127] B. D'Onofrio et al., "Paternal Age at Childbearing and Offspring Psychiatric and Academic Morbidity," *JAMA Psychiatry* 71, no. 4 (2014): 432-438; S. Sandin et al., "Autism risk associated with parental age and with increasing difference in age between the parents," *Molecular Psychiatry* (June 9, 2015): doi:10.1038/mp.2015.70.
[128] B. D'Onofrio et al., "Paternal Age at Childbearing," 432-438.
[129] American Society of Reproductive Medicine and Society for Assisted Reproductive Technology, "Recommendations for gamete and embryo donation," 48; Health Canada, "Health Canada Directive: Technical Requirements for Therapeutic Donor Insemination," (2000), http://www.hc-sc.gc.ca/dhp-mps/alt_formats/hpfb-dgpsa/pdf/prodpharma/semen-sperme_directive-eng.pdf.

[130] American Society of Reproductive Medicine, "Recommendations for gamete and embryo donation," 48.
[131] Health Canada, "Health Canada Directive: Technical Requirements for Therapeutic Donor Insemination," (2000), http://www.hc-sc.gc.ca/dhp-mps/alt_formats/hpfb-dgpsa/pdf/prodpharma/semen-sperme_directive-eng.pdf.
[132] ASRM, "Third-party Reproduction: Sperm, egg, and embryo donation and surrogacy. A Guide for Patients, Revised 2012," https://www.asrm.org/uploadedFiles/ASRM_Con10t/Resources/Patient_Resources/Fact_Sheets_and_Info_Booklets/thirdparty.pdf.
[133] Directive 2004/23/EC of the European Parliament and of the Council, "On setting standards of quality and safety for the donation, procurement, testing, processing, preservation, storage and distribution of human tissues and cells," *Official Journal of the European Union* (2004): 48. http://eur-lex.europa.eu/legal-content/EN/TXT/?uri=celex:32004L0023.
[134] American Society of Reproductive Medicine, "Recommendations for gamete and embryo donation"; Health Canada, "Health Canada Directive."; Commission Directive 2006/17/EC. Official Journal of the European Union Anex III, (2006): 38. http://eur-lex.europa.eu/legal-con10t/EN/TXT/?uri=CELEX%3A32006L0017; U.S. Food and Drug Administration Electronic Code of Federal Regulations. Subpart C 1271.75; 1271.80; 1271.85, http://www.accessdata.fda.gov/scripts/cdrh/cfdocs/cfcfr/CFRSearch.cfm?CFRPart=1271&showFR=1&subpartNode=21:8.0.1.5.57.3.
[135] Health Canada, "Health Canada Directive."
[136] ASRM, "Third-party Reproduction: Sperm, egg, and embryo donation and surrogacy. A Guide for Patients, Revised 2012," http://www.reproductivefacts.org/uploadedFiles/ASRM_Content/Resources/Patient_Resources/Fact_Sheets_and_Info_Booklets/thirdparty.pdf; American Association of Tissue Banks (2008), "State Requirements for Tissue Bank Licensure, Registration or Certification," (November 2008), http://www.aatb.org/State-Requirements-for-Tissue-Bank-Licensure-Registration-or-Certification.
[137] Health Canada, "Health Canada Directive."
[138] Kamal Ahuja, "Is the UK sperm donor shortage a myth?" *Bionews Online* 802, (May 18, 2015), http://www.bionews.org.uk/page_526622.asp?hlight=Is+the+UK+sperm+donor+shortage+a+myth%3F.
[139] Fairfax Cryobank, "Why choose Fairfax?" Accessed on January 3, 2016, http://www.fairfaxcryobank.ca/.
[140] G. Benagiano et al., "Italian Constitutional Court removes the prohibition on gamete donation in Italy," *Reproductive BioMedicine Online* 29, no. 6 (2014): 662-664.
[141] B. Bay et al., "Danish sperm donors across three decades: motivations and attitudes," *Fertility and Sterility* 101, no. 1 (2014): 253.
[142] M. Daudin et al., "Sperm cryopreservation in adolescents and young adults with cancer: results of the French national sperm banking network (CECOS)," *Fertility and Sterility* 102, no. 2 (2015): 478-486. e1.

143 Human Fertilisation and Embryology Authority, "Conceived on or after 1 April 2005," http://www.hfea.gov.uk/5554.html.
144 B. Bay et al., "Danish sperm donors."
145 Victoria Assisted Reproductive Treatment Authority (VARTA), "Regulation," accessed December 22, 2015, https://www.varta.org.au/regulation/legislation-and-guideline-overview.
146 Fairfax Cryobank, accessed December 22, 2015, https://fairfaxcryobank.com/us/.38 S. Isaksson et al., "It takes two to tango: Information sharing with offspring among heterosexual parents following identity-release sperm donation," Human Reproduction 3, no. 1 (2016):125-132.
147 S. Isaksson et al., "It takes two to tango: Information sharing with offspring among heterosexual parents following identity-release sperm donation," *Human Reproduction* 3, no. 1 (2016):125-132.
148 B. Bay et al., "Danish sperm donors."
149 S. Zadeh, T. Freeman, and S. Golombok, "Absence or presence? Complexities in the donor narratives of single mothers using sperm donation," Human Reproduction 31, no. 1 (2016): 117-124.
150 Government of Canada, Justice, "Assisted Human Reproduction Act," (2004), http://laws-lois.justice.gc.ca/eng/acts/A-13.4/FullText.html.
151 Human Fertilisation and Embryology Authority, *SEED Report. A report on the Human Fertilisation & Embryology Authority's review of sperm, egg and embryo donation in the United Kingdom*, (2005), 13.
152 H. Bissessar, "Donor Sperm: Why the high cost low supply," Creating Families (2010): 10-13.
153 S. Parnell, "Australia's assisted reproduction fueled by imported US sperm," September 14, 2015, accessed December 27, 2015, https://www.geneticliteracyproject.org/2015/09/14/australias-assisted-reproduction-fueled-by-imported-us-sperm/.
154 Kamal, K. Ahuja, "Patient pressure: is the tide of cross-border reproductive care beginning to turn?" reproduced in *Biomed Online* 30, (2015): 447-450.
155 Human Fertilisation and Embryology Authority, "HFEA agree new policies."
156 National Gamete Donation Trust, "Sperm Donor," accessed December 27, 2015, http://www.ngdt.co.uk/sperm-donor.
157 A. Ochert, "UK national sperm bank only has nine donors," *BioNews Online* 818, (2015).
158 Kamal Ahuja, "Is the UK sperm donor shortage a myth?"
159 M. Daudin et al., "Sperm cryopreservation in adolescents and young adults with cancer: results of the French national sperm banking network (CECOS)," *Fertility and Sterility* 102, no. 2 (2015): 478-486.e1.
160 D. Le Lannou, B. Lobel, and Y. Chambon, "Sperm Banks and Donor Recruitment in France," *Human Artificial Insemination and Semen Preservation*, eds., D. Georges and P.David, (Paris: Plenum Press, 1979).
161 Agence de la biomédecine, "Assisted reproductive technology," (2013), accessed December 27, 2015. http://www.agence-biomedecine.fr/Assisted-reproductive-technology?lang=fr

---

[162] I. Ferrara, R. Balet, and J.G. Grudzinskas, "Intrauterine insemination with frozen donor sperm. Pregnancy outcome in relation to age and ovarian stimulation regime," *Human Reproduction*, (2002), Vol.17 (9), 2320-2324; S. Allamaneni, I. Bandaranayake, and A. Agarwal, "Use of semen quality scores to predict pregnancy rates in couples undergoing intrauterine insemination with donor sperm," *Fertility and Sterility* 82, no. 3 (2004): 606-611.

[163] ASRM, "Age and Fertility - A Guide for Patients" (2012), http://www.reproductivefacts.org/; A. Cheung et al., "SOGC Clinical Practice Guideline - Advanced Reproductive Age and Fertility," JOGC (2011): 1165-1175.

[164] N. Carroll and J. Palmer, "A comparison of intrauterine versus intracervical insemination in fertile single women," *Fertility and Sterility* 74, no. 4 (2001): 656-666; D. Chavkin et al., "Donor Sperm Insemination Cycles: Are two inseminations better than one?" *Journal of Andrology* 33, no. 3 (2012): 375-379; D.E. Besselink et al., "Cervical insemination versus intra-uterine insemination of donor sperm for subfertility," *Cochrane Database of Systematic Reviews* no. 2 (Apr 16, 2008), doi:10.1002/14651858.CD000317.pub3.

[165] P.A.L. Kop et al., "Intrauterine insemination or intracervical insemination with cryopreserved donor sperm in the natural cycle: A cohort study," *Human Reproduction* 30 no. 3 (2015): 603-607, doi:10.1093/humrep/dev004.

[166] S. Corbett et al., "Access to fertility services for lesbian women in Canada," *Fertility and Sterility* 100, no. 4 (2013) 1077-1080; L. Ross, L.S. Steele, and R.I. Epstein, "Lesbian and bisexual women's recommendations for improving the provision of assisted reproductive technology services," *Fertility and Sterility* 86, no. 3 (2006): 735-738; ASRM The Ethics Committee of the American Society for Reproductive Medicine, "Access to fertility treatments by gays, lesbians, and unmarried persons," *Fertility and Sterility* 92, no. 4 (2009): 1170-1193.

[167] Repromed, http://www.repromed.ca/home_insemination.html; Fairfax Cryobank,https://fairfaxcryobank.com/us/ordering-shipping-faqs#whenarrive; Xytex Cryo International, https://www.xytex.com/sperm-donor-bank-patient/sperm-donor-bank-patient-faq.cfm.

[168] Cryos International, https://dk.cryosinternational.com/resources/questions-answers/.

[169] Human Fertilisation and Embryology Authority, "Procuring, processing and transporting gametes and embryos, HFEA Guidance: Home Insemination," http://www.hfea.gov.uk/503.html#guidanceSection4638.

[170] D. Chavkin et al., "Donor Sperm Insemination Cycles," 375-379.

[171] S. Zarek et al., "Single-donor and double-donor sperm intrauterine insemination cycles: does double intrauterine insemination increase clinical pregnancy rates?" *Fertility and Sterility* 102 (2014): 739-43.

[172] National Gamete Donation Trust, "Sperm Donor," accessed December 27, 2015, http://www.ngdt.co.uk/sperm-donor.

[173] Victoria Assisted Reproductive Treatment Authority (VARTA), "Regulation."

[174] Ibid.

[175] American Society of Reproductive Medicine, "Recommendations for gamete and embryo donation," 48.

[176] P. Janssens et al., "Evolving minimum standards in responsible international sperm donor offspring quota," *Reproductive BioMedicine Online* 30, no. 6 (2015): 568-580.
[177] Fairfax Cryobank, "Why Choose Fairfax"; California Cryobank, accessed December 27, 2015, http://www.cryobank.com/Services/Pricing/#DonorSemen_box; Cryos International, accessed December28, 2015. https://dk.cryosinternational.com/donor-sperm/the-donors/
[178] Fairfax Cryobank, "Sperm Donor FAQs," https://beaspermdonor.com/spermdonorfaqs.shtml; Xytex Corporation, "Become a Donor FAQ," https://www.xytex.com/sperm-donor-bank-become-donor/sperm-donor-faq.cfm; Cryos USA, "Sperm Donor Application Orlando," https://usa.cryosinternational.com/become-a-donor/become-a-sperm-donor/donor-application/online-application-orlando/.
[179] Donor Sibling Registry, accessed January 5, 2016, https://www.donorsiblingregistry.com/about-dsr/history-and-mission.
[180] Donor Conception Network, http://www.dcnetwork.org/.
[181] Kamal Ahuja, "Is the UK sperm donor shortage a myth?"
[182] G. Benagiano et al., "Italian Constitutional Court removes the prohibition on gamete donation in Italy," *Reproductive Biomedicine Online* 29, no. 6 (2014): 662-664.
[183] Agence de la biomédecine, "Assisted reproductive technology."

Chapter 7: Egg Donation and Surrogacy

The Greatest Leap of Faith: Becoming a Sole Parent

So, where to begin—

Ever since I was a little girl, I had always wanted to be a mom. Never did it cross my mind that I would have difficulty getting there.

Growing up within a large, extended, Italian family, I took for granted that these things just happened. It worked that way for my dozens of cousins, so why was I having such difficulty? Ok, so most were in their early to mid-twenties, but I was climbing my career ladder when I was that age. Besides, there was lots of time to think about having children; I wasn't in a rush.

Time sure flies! All of a sudden, I was thirty-nine. Hmmm, if I was serious about having children, I had better start to make a plan. However, I wasn't married nor did I have a partner.

I went off the birth control pill (BCP) to start regulating my cycles. Apparently, they were all over the place, and after a few months I went to see my family doctor. I hadn't a worry; I was in great health. Blood tests showed that I had very high FSH levels and I was diagnosed with Premature Ovarian Failure (POF). Basically, I had no eggs but the cooker was still good. I had been on the BCP for a dozen years so my periods were super light but ran like clockwork. I was then referred to a fertility specialist. We ran tests after tests, tried different medications, alternative supplements, and I had every procedure (or so it felt like) under the sun. My cycle did not want to show up for this party! Months had turned into three years and I still honestly believed that it would all come together. Boy was I naïve.

The day came where I was in the doctor's office and it was becoming clear that having a baby wasn't in the cards for me. I was forty-two and running out of time, literally. But if I really, really, wanted to do this I would have to consider other options. Adoption? Surrogacy? Egg donation? Like yesterday!

I took a couple of months off "fertility talk" then started researching adoption. I went to a seminar for intended parents. The testimonial couples were very encouraging with their stories and advice even though the process was long, but not guaranteed. However, the more research and questions I asked, the more it became very clear that a single person isn't the ideal "family" that a birth mother would choose for the child she is about to give up. There are no guarantees you will get a child, you could potentially wait indefinitely, and even if you are chosen to be the parent, there is always the chance the birth mother may change her mind. I was forty-two, nearing forty-three at this point, and "indefinitely" wasn't the route for me. And surrogacy didn't really make sense in my situation. Egg donation was it. I guess. It took a few more months to really come to grips with the reality that I could not have a baby. I had no eggs. How was this even possible? I was healthier at this age than I'd ever been, and in the best shape of my life! Yet my body had failed me. I was sad, angry, depressed, and I started to resent mothers who just sneezed and ended up pregnant.

After much soul searching, I decided that even though I'd never have a baby of my own, perhaps I could still be a mom. For me, I didn't want to be staring fifty in the face, knowing that it was too late. I didn't want to look back and regret not trying. If I tried and it didn't work, then at least I'd know I had done everything I could. I made another appointment with the fertility specialist to talk more about the egg donation process and where to go for help. She talked me through it and, upon leaving, gave me a few brochures from agencies here in Canada, as well as international agencies. I left her office feeling more positive, happy, even excited, and I looked forward to reading more.

I sent out a couple of emails, one to a Toronto-based agency, and the other to an overseas agency with an office in Toronto. I didn't hear from the first agency for a number of weeks. But the overseas agency was very quick to respond and I felt good now that the ice was broken. I also learned that when it came time for egg collection and embryo transfer, it would be done by their doctors at their clinic, internationally, not with my own trusted doctors. This definitely frightened me and I didn't understand the logistics yet, but I just kept reminding myself what could be waiting for me at the end of the journey.

Over the next few months, I asked them absolutely everything under the sun about the steps towards mamma hood. They even went so far as to set up a special personal meeting with the founder/director of the agency as he was going to be in my area for a conference. We met for a casual coffee, and armed with my list of questions, I asked and he answered—every question, kindly and thoroughly. I left knowing that I was ready to make the final decision. The next step was to confirm my commitment to this process—IVF via egg donor. Wow!

After I sent a message stating my commitment, it was full steam ahead! The agency has very strict parameters for their egg donors. After they told me the guidelines, they sent me a few donor profiles to review. These came with one or two photos, and a list of physical characteristics, parents and sibling's physical characteristics, age, profession, whether or not the donor had prior successful donations, blood type, medical information, any allergies, genetic conditions, or metabolic disorders. In my case, they sent donor sperm profiles too, which followed the same guidelines.

It took a few days but I finally chose an egg donor. We shared some of the same physical characteristics, interests and even had similar professions. After a few days, the agency confirmed with me that the donor I chose was available and she would start her fertility treatments in preparation for egg collection. Woo-hoo!!

Egg donor. Check. Sperm donor. Check. Then the agency sent me a medical protocol. There were a number of procedures, medicines, and supplements that I would need to have prior to egg collection. We had to make sure my body was ready and willing to accept an embryo. Besides, I had only enough funds to do this once so I needed to cross all the t's and dot all the i's.

The protocol was very thorough and a bit complex. Way too complex for me to even begin to wrap my head around. However, the agency team was in constant contact with me and my home fertility physician. They managed all the logistical timelines and scheduling of absolutely everything. They would email me what step would come next, where I needed to be, and what day to be there. I was never stressed, confused, or overwhelmed.

About six to eight weeks after the medical protocol, my donor was ready for her egg collection; however, one of my medical procedures came back with non-optimal findings. This resulted in a delay in my embryo-transfer scheduling. My travel plans were cancelled and I was referred to another specialist to perform a very specific medical procedure. The waiting period to see this specialist was at least three months.

My stomach dropped to my feet. I didn't have three months! Every day counted. We decided to go ahead with the egg collection and fertilization of the embryos and then they were to be frozen for me until transfer was more favorable. A few days after the collection and fertilization, I was given the most awesome news that there were six very strong embryos!

Although only two are allowed to be transferred at one time, there were six shots at a viable pregnancy! After venting my frustration to a friend, regarding the major hiccup of postponement, an almost miracle happened. Whether a stroke of luck or possibly a divine intervention, that friend knew a friend who worked with a doctor who did these exact procedures. I was scheduled for the procedure in three weeks and the results were in favor of embryo transfer. I was elated.

After another month of hormone patches, medications, and monitoring, I was finally ready to travel to the clinic overseas for my embryo transfer. My home physician, her nurses, and staff did an outstanding job of coordinating with the overseas agency during a very long six months of prepping my body to get to this stage. Looking back, it was almost May when I started with the hormone preparations and now we were in the final month, because at the end of October I was booked to fly. This was it; I was going to do this!

Aside from the coordination with my physician and her staff, the overseas agency took care of everything from booking my flights, to accommodation and transfers. They even provided a professional, and very personable, escort to accompany me to and from the airport, to take me to the clinic for my pre-op check-up, and just to keep me company.

I had five days away in total. The first was my travel day. The second day was the pre-op check-up. Embryo transfer was on day three, followed by rest and relaxation!!!!! Day four was an organized personal tour of some tourist attractions and a great lunch with my escort. Day five, I travelled back home.

The entire time I was blessed with being able to maintain positivity. At no point did I believe that this would not work. This was my shot, and I could see the light at the end of that long tunnel. Day after day, that light was shining brighter and brighter. They call it the "two-week wait," because after embryo transfer, your next blood test isn't for two weeks. I went about my daily business like nothing had happened. The two weeks went by quickly and I went for my blood tests. The results indicated that there might be a pregnancy, and I was to repeat the test again in two days. If this one had numbers that doubled, then a pregnancy had been achieved. And that's exactly what happened. At six weeks, I had my first ultrasound, which confirmed the pregnancy. Although there was no heartbeat yet, the pregnancy was confirmed!!!!!

I started to read online and after about a day, I quickly stopped. I learned that there's a lot of women that really obsess and stress over this stuff. I took a different approach and just believed that what would be, would be. It was medically out of my hands at this point, and it was in my and my new, long-awaited pregnancy's best interest for me to just stay positive, keep stresses at bay, and keep my eye on the prize. Once my pregnancy was deemed viable around twelve to fourteen weeks, I was referred to an obstetrician who continued the process with amazing care.

My eye was on that prize for thirty-nine weeks and, at forty-four years of age, I gave birth to a beautiful baby girl. Looking back, my pregnancy was not without worry; however, it was almost as if I had a guardian angel to keep me positive and calm. Perhaps my dad was watching over me and my little one—he never got to meet his granddaughter. Whatever it was, I am so happy and blessed to have been given the opportunity to go through this process.

My four remaining embryos were frozen for my future use. When my daughter turned two, I had to make the gut-wrenching decision to keep them for another year, unfreeze them and let them perish, or donate them to intended parents.

As much as I wanted to have another child, to try for a sibling for my daughter, I was now forty-six and on my own. If I had a partner, you bet, I wouldn't have given it a second thought. Letting them perish turned my stomach, especially knowing what infertility issues I had gone through. The obvious choice was to donate four very healthy embryos. I made it a condition upon donation that I be notified if a live birth resulted and that there would be the option for my daughter to meet her sibling should she want to when she turned eighteen. This gave me hope, happiness and contentment.

If I could give someone advice as to whether or not to use an egg donor, I would definitely be pro-donor. You don't even realize the amount of stress weighing you down when you're stuck in that thought of never being able to have your own child.

Once you've made the decision to pursue egg donation, that weight is lifted automatically. My head may know that it wasn't my egg that gave me the gift of a child, but my heart doesn't care. She is 100 percent mine and I love her with all of my being.

Timea Belej-Rak, M.D.

Our Fertility Story

I always knew I was going to have a family one day, but I never knew it would take this long to become pregnant. You always hear others tell you they are having a baby but you never hear the story of how long it may have taken them to get pregnant. You buy a house, get married, and have children. At least that's what I thought would happen to me. But unfortunately, that was not in my cards. It took me and my husband four years to conceive. And it wasn't done the natural way. In fact, it wasn't even our own eggs or sperm.

Our fertility journey has seemed like a long road to success. Not to mention thousands and thousands of dollars. Why us?

Why me?

Everyone else was having babies before me when I thought I would be the first. What was wrong with me? What did I do to deserve this? These are the thoughts that would go through my head.

It all started back in 2011. One month after we got married, we decided to start a family. I was so excited to start this journey and thought I'd be pregnant within three months. Three months came and went and no baby. Another month went by, and another and another. Eight months passed and still no positive pregnancy test. I cannot tell you how tired I was of seeing that line say negative.

We thought we might need to go to a fertility specialist, so we got on the waiting list and after two months we had our first appointment with the fertility doctor. I had to do many, many blood tests and three cycle monitorings with Clomid where they just wanted to see how my body acted. I was on that medication for way too long and it did nothing for me. I still wasn't pregnant. I was starting to become a bit frustrated because I thought they would "cure" whatever was wrong with me. Then they found out that I had low ovarian reserve. I went home that day and did some research and it turned out I couldn't do anything to prevent it. My husband got tested also and all seemed normal. So back to the clinic I went for another cycle monitoring, but this time on a different medication. Frankly, I just seemed like a number as this was a big clinic and they just seemed to do the same treatment on me. This went on for another six months, and by then I decided I needed to try another clinic.

Clinic number two made me feel so much more comfortable and the nurses were great. They really were there to help and support me through this tough journey. My husband got tested again and all seemed normal. Finally, a clinic that didn't just put me on Clomid. I had one cycle monitoring and then went straight to intrauterine insemination (IUI). A step up. I thought this could be it. This could really happen. Then I got that dreaded phone call at the end of the cycle: "We are so sorry to tell you but your pregnancy test came out negative." I could not believe it. I thought this would work.

So onto another cycle of IUI and still the same result. We tried one more time and once again another negative blood test. So we met with the fertility doctor to go over next steps which was of course, in vitro fertilization (IVF). Well this just had to work; IVF was known to solve everyone's problems.

Or so I thought. It was also an expense we didn't expect. I'm sure everyone who has gone through this can relate to the emotions and the sacrifices your body experiences. Each time I injected myself with the medication, I felt it was going to make my body work overtime and get things going again. But my situation was a bit different from others; my body just didn't want to produce more than one follicle. How could this be? I had injected myself with something that was supposed to produce many, many follicles. Going over our results with the nurses we decided it was best to cancel this IVF cycle. All that for nothing, it seemed. So we did another month of injections and another IVF cycle, only to have the same outcome. Then we tried it once more, hoping this time I would produce more follicles. I had about two good ones. Still nothing compared to the average ten to twenty. I will never forget the phone call I had on my way to work. The fertility doctor called me to go over my results and see if we were going to proceed. He said the chances of this resulting in a pregnancy were slim and he thought the next step was donor eggs. "Donor eggs?!" I thought.

This word seemed foreign to me and hurtful. How could a healthy, thirty-three-year-old be going the donor egg route!

I acted polite on the phone and said I would have to discuss it with my husband. We decided to cancel the cycle. I was bawling my eyes out on the way to work that day, as I couldn't fathom the idea of having someone else's eggs and it not being "my baby." It didn't seem right. That night my husband and I talked it over and thought we needed to take a break.

We'd been doing two years of fertility treatments with zero results. I got back into fitness and was even going to do a fitness competition because I had started to feel good about myself again. I put my mind off having babies and focused on enjoying life and being married. We got a new house, a new car, and a new puppy and that seemed to put our minds at ease. But after a while, reality sank back in and I wanted to try again. Life didn't seem complete. So my husband and I talked it over and decided to try another clinic and another doctor's advice. Maybe this time an IVF cycle would actually work and maybe they would use some other technique on me.

We met with the doctor at clinic number three in 2014. He seemed nice and would even call us from home at night to talk about his strategy and the clinic. He was surprised that the other clinic would even mention using donor eggs. He didn't think this would be something for us so we got tested again and my husband's sperm all came back normal. I did one cycle monitoring before we did an IVF cycle. I knew the result of my follicles for IVF would be low but I was hoping the clinic would look at my past results and try something different. He gave me a higher dose of the medication and another injection. I thought, OK, this has got to work. I produced two follicles and that was it. Nothing had changed.

So my husband and I decided we were going to go for this IVF cycle. It was all or nothing. I could have a good egg in that follicle that would fertilize and implant. All you need is one. So we did egg retrieval and my egg was no good. The doctor said that I would have to think of using an egg donor.

I remember feeling like a brick wall had hit me. Seeing my husband afterwards and telling him the news was hard. I just wanted to cry in bed all day. To top this off, it was almost Christmas time. My husband and I did not like this clinic at all, and their nurses were nowhere near the ones at the second clinic. There wasn't even a follow up phone call to discuss our next steps. We were on our own again.

Wasting no time, I did some online research for donor clinics and my husband and I came to the realization that we had to do this if we wanted a baby. We had tried everything and I wasn't getting any younger. I emailed the second clinic and they said they were in contact with an egg donation agency. It looked legit online and had great reviews, so I emailed and their coordinator emailed me right away to set up a phone interview with the general manager. We spent almost an hour talking about what their program had to offer.

He was very sincere and helpful and gave me details about what I would be going through, how the program worked, and what the processes were. I was very excited when I got off the phone and gave the news to my husband. He was happy with what he read but there was only one thing. This was another expense. Luckily, we have a generous family and were able to take the rest out of our savings, but it was well worth it.

I read about the pregnancy rates and felt confident about using donor eggs so we started the process of donor selection. First, we had to send in a detailed copy of what we were looking for in the donor and then the coordinator sent us ones that were compatible. I was quite impressed with the first donor. She was pretty, had a good education, and had in-depth health screenings. They even had her family history and background which was important to us. We received more donor profiles and they were all so good, but one in particular stood out from the rest. She looked like me, was young, and had previous successful donor pregnancies. She also had a great background; she was in business and her parents were a doctor and teacher. How much better could you get? I got pretty excited after picking her. We told our families, who had been very supportive. My parents, who hadn't thought the donors would be this good, were quite impressed. Once we picked our donor we just had to wait until she did her IVF cycle. The general manager at the egg donation agency was so good at communicating to us about how things were going in Europe, where our donor lived. He always made himself available.

We were told our embryos were ready to be shipped and I was so excited. When they arrived, we were surprised to discover that only four had reached the blastocyst stage, but that our donor had produced fifteen good quality eggs. Then another red flag went up: my husband's sperm would not fertilize properly. The agency was concerned and used the rest of his sperm on other eggs that were previously banked but still nothing would fertilize. My husband couldn't believe this. He thought it had to be wrong, as all this time he had been told his sperm were normal. The agency found out that they appeared good, but when it came to fertilization, they just wouldn't take. Because of this and because the results of the embryos shipped weren't what we expected, the general manager said he would do another cycle with the same donor without charge. They were concerned for us and very interested in this case, as they had not seen anything like it before. We were so thankful and that is when it hit home that they really cared and were there to help us get pregnant.

On the general manager's recommendation, my husband got a FISH test done to see if there was something wrong with the genetic makeup of the sperm, but it came back normal. We are baffled about what the story is, but we won't ever really know. We decided to use my husband's sperm on half of the donor's eggs, and donor sperm on the other half. His didn't fertilize any of them but it was a risk we wanted to take.

The donor sperm had no problem. The agency had given us some sperm donor profiles and like the egg donors, they were very detailed. We choose one and waited until everything was shipped back. I must say that this whole process is so amazing. Our donor produced fourteen mature eggs and the rest of the embryos were shipped to my home fertility clinic.

I cannot believe that someone gets the embryos, and flies them back to where I live. It's astonishing. It takes a lot of organization to do this. It was November 2015 when they implanted two good quality embryos into me. After four years, I had never gotten to this stage so it was very exciting and I was very hopeful. I took a few days off work to just relax and watch movies. I felt something different inside me and I didn't want to say anything to anyone but I was sure I was feeling implantation. It was a great feeling.

I was so nervous the day I had to do my blood pregnancy test. I will never forget the two words they told me later that day: "You're pregnant." My heart literally stopped. Those words seemed so foreign to me. I was the happiest girl ever! I remember getting off the phone, kneeling over and crying happy tears. I was in disbelief. So this is how it feels. I called my husband right away and we shared the excitement. And then of course I had to make the call to my parents and they were over the moon for us. We shared our news over Christmas 2015 with family and it was the best Christmas ever. We are expecting a baby girl and I have had the best pregnancy. I look at my belly each day and watch it grow, and I am no longer afraid to say I had to use donor eggs and donor sperm. Having a baby has been my dream for quite some time, and I can't thank the agency enough; it is a place where dreams really do come true.

I Never Planned For This!—Egg Donation and Surrogacy;

by David Sher, CEO, ELITE IVF

"I never planned for this!" is probably the first thing that goes through your mind when your physician says that you need to use egg donation or surrogacy. It's something you never imagined, wanted, or even knew existed as an option for your own reproduction. It reminds me of when I started in the field of IVF.

I was approached by a group of investors in 2002 and asked to create a business plan for a global IVF agency. Eggs. Sperm. Mix them up and create embryos to "transfer" to a uterus. It sounded like science fiction and although I knew what each was, the discussion and focus on them as independent entities that come together to create life seemed surreal. By the time I was able to wrap my mind around those concepts I was told, "Hey now, if the eggs are not viable, then you need to get a donor for those eggs or sperm." It was enough to send me reaching for a stiff drink.

I never planned for this as a career choice—helping couples with egg donation. But, I was sure that they never planned for it either, so at least we were in the same boat. How could I add value to someone who needs egg donation, I wondered?

About a year later, I concluded my research and reflection on that question and launched what is today a dynamic, continuously growing (fortunately for me, but a sad reflection of the infertility reality in our world) global services company.

I approached the subject matter from a patient's perspective: How would I want to be treated by the "system" of solutions available to me if I were told that I needed egg donation in order to achieve my family-planning goals?

Surveying the landscape, I realized that the world of fertility, and specifically egg donation, was loaded with inefficiencies and imperfections that were making patients' lives miserable, or at best less than optimal. It was 2004 and Canadian legislation had just turned against egg donation.

Overnight it dictated to fertility patients that egg donation was no longer legal in Canada! Well, it was legal, but not if you were a voluntary egg donor who was willing to help an intended parent couple, and in return for your time and effort receive compensation. That transaction in Canada would now constitute a crime, both for the donor and the recipient.

I never planned for this! A Canadian egg donor could donate to a couple, but could not receive any compensation for it. Yeah right, this would really be productive in terms of attracting voluntary candidates, I thought. Predictably, egg donation in Canada turned into a desert landscape overnight, when the rains that fed the earth—the donors—vanished. Only an arid landscape, disturbed by the occasional tumbleweed, remained.

Tumbleweeds in this metaphor were altruistic egg donors, those most angelic of angels who were willing to donate their eggs for no compensation at all. However, with demand by intended parents totally overwhelming supply, those few tumbleweeds were as practical as they are in the desert (not very) in helping to meet the needs of people seeking egg donors.

A solution was needed and that solution became obvious—outsource egg donation abroad! Sounds great and even exciting at first, but after the initial exhilaration, when you start thinking of how to go about it, you quickly realize that it's worse than you ever imagined!

Fortunately, I did plan for this, but only because I had the luxury of time and no pressure. My investors let me explore the field of egg donation for about one year to find the right formula to help patients who were facing one of life's most daunting personal challenges.

The solution was to find egg donors around the world, standardize their screening, and make them accessible to Canadian patients who needed their donations of eggs. Next, I created a very personalized management process to help cushion the patient against the many pitfalls involved in undertaking a cross-border fertility treatment involving egg donation.

The tailored, all-inclusive "treatment package," as it became known, included everything you would need in order to complete your egg donation treatment with us. Without it, there were so many moving parts and issues to consider that the potential to get lost in the minutiae would be overwhelming. Instead, we would make all this stress and uncertainty vanish, or at least minimize it to the greatest degree possible, so you could focus on yourself and your physical and emotional preparation. We would provide this package for one all-inclusive fee, which would allow you to control and predict your total treatment cost rather than just one aspect of it, thus reducing the anxiety of the unknown and shifting control back into your hands.

Treatment Package

- Recruitment and matching with an egg donor,
- medical preparation of the intended mother in Canada for the imminent donor egg-conceived, embryo transfer abroad,
- entire cost of the egg donation cycle abroad (donor reimbursement, donor medication, travel, IVF cycle, and all clinical work including donor screening),

- return flight tickets for the intended parents to the destination clinic and country where the egg donation would take place,
- a week's stay at a five-star hotel, all local transportation from the airport to the hotel, the clinic and back, as needed for treatment,
- everything at the recipient's home clinic leading up to the departure abroad, and the early pregnancy monitoring until the pregnancy blood test at home upon the return of the patient.

Case Management Team

Surrounding this entire experience was a case management team that would manage the entire treatment process for you from the moment you contacted us for an inquiry until the end of your first trimester. The team included a patient intake coordinator (helping you navigate the range of options available with our company), a medical coordinator (working 24/7 with you on all of your medical issues, and directing you in writing and over the phone each step of the way), a logistics coordinator (making all of the flight and hotel arrangements for you so you could concentrate on your treatment), an administrator (providing and maintaining the records, contracts, and invoices for your treatment package), and finally, an on-site patient coordinator (greeting you abroad at the airport with a private car and chauffer, assisting you through the one week requisite stay, taking you to and from appointments, and even going with you into the procedure room if desired). This allowed us to manage the experience from beginning to end, and shoulder the burden of stress that going abroad for an egg donation treatment entailed. In my research, I realized that there was a need for managing the gap that inevitably existed between the home country of the intended parents and the destination country where their donor was waiting to provide them with her eggs. There were so many pitfalls involved. If you tried to just "do it yourself" you would have an exceptional amount of additional stress, unpredictable costs, and a lack of accountability by the medical professionals involved. Most importantly, you would experience great loneliness trying to navigate through the myriad of issues, likely resulting in a considerable delay in treatment and a lot of aggravation.

I never planned for this, but my vision struck a chord and provided a beautiful and harmonious solution for Canadian patients seeking egg donation. Very quickly we expanded the service offering to other countries, and today I manage a global fertility services company that provides this solution to patients not just from Canada, but from around the world. We have also expanded our donor recruitment to encompass multiple regions, including the USA, Europe, Mexico, and Panama, offering a variety of ethnicities that can meet the donor matching needs of almost any type of patient. We have many different ethnicities represented, including East Indian and Chinese.

Vitrification

For over a decade, if you were our patient and had decided to proceed with egg donation, you had a lot of choice in terms of where to go for treatment (Europe, USA, Mexico, Panama, etc.) but only one way to do it—fresh egg donation. This has been a great solution for our Canadian patients since 2004, as we have seen hundreds become parents though the process, not once but even twice or three times when they came back to repeat it for siblings using the same egg donor.

Since then, significant changes have taken place including one of the most profound—a freezing technology known as vitrification, or "fast freezing." Previously, eggs or embryos were frozen through a process known as "slow freeze." This process produced thaw survival rates of about 60 percent.

Eggs did not survive the thawing process, so it was mainly applicable to the freezing of embryos. With the arrival of vitrification, thaw survival rates went up to almost 100 percent, rendering the need for doing things "fresh" unnecessary.

We have known about vitrification since 2007, but even though we made every effort to convince Canadian IVF clinics to use this ground-breaking technology, they weren't interested: "Why fix what's not broken." Apparently, the infamous attitude of Canadians towards risk aversion has been given free rein in the field of Canadian fertility, in spite of mounting scientific evidence and our own experience with successful vitrification at our clinics in Spain and Mexico.

Ironically, the Mexican clinics were years ahead of Canadian ones since they were more open to experimentation, and were validating new technologies before their Canadian colleagues. It did not help that some Canadian physicians looked down upon Mexican physicians and anything that was being done "down there in Mexico."

They were wrong. Around 2011 we heard that even the US clinics were recognizing vitrification as "non-experimental."

We saw this as the green light to push ahead with some very innovative plans. We sent Canada's finest lab directors to inspect our IVF labs in Mexico and Europe, and to undergo some training with their Mexican counterparts. When they returned, the Canadians said that they were ready to start using vitrification in their clinics, and the age of "frozen eggs" was born. We were the first to bring frozen eggs to Canada, which meant that flying to a destination clinic outside of Canada wasn't necessary anymore. A patient would select a donor with us as they always did, and then we would stimulate, collect and freeze that donor's eggs. The eggs would be shipped to Canada where the patient's clinic would thaw them, fertilize them, and do the embryo transfer. A new way of doing egg donation was born!

Unfortunately, not all was rosy. In our pilot program with one of Canada's leading IVF clinics, most of the patients did get pregnant but the experiment uncovered a major flaw with frozen donor eggs. Our patients would receive twelve eggs, but after thawing, instead of getting an average of five to six blastocysts (embryos that have spent five days developing in the IVF lab after initial fertilization), we would see between one and two.

Fortunately, that was all patients needed to get pregnant, but from a clinical and professional perspective, we were having cold sweats at night. What if those few embryos do not achieve a pregnancy? There was no back up. There were not enough embryos in reserve to help the patient carry on with repeated attempts. There were three particularly agonizing patient cases where our repeated efforts (using upwards of thirty to forty eggs per patient) did not result in viable blastocysts.

In our desperation to help patients, we decided to change our approach; we froze semen in Toronto and shipped it to our center in Europe. Using the same egg donors, we repeated their egg donation cycles, but this time, instead of freezing the donor eggs, we fertilized the eggs when they were fresh.

The results were drastically different, and better. We suddenly achieved the five to six blastocysts per patient that we would normally expect to see. So, we froze the embryos and shipped them back to Canada. In each case, one blastocyst embryo was thawed back in Canada and transferred to the uterus of the patient, resulting in an ongoing pregnancy and a birth.

This was a turning point in our history, and possibly in how treatments were being done in Canada. Our signature egg donation program was born—the frozen embryo program!

Frozen Embryo Program

Today, the frozen embryo program is our recommended program for egg donation. We create frozen embryos from donor eggs abroad, using a fresh egg donation cycle, but we do the embryo transfer back in Canada. It is the culmination of twelve years of work, and everything we have learned to date, packaged into an amazing way of doing egg donation.

Now you don't need to travel abroad. You are still welcome to do it if you want an excuse for a vacation, but by using our frozen embryo program, you can stay at home while we bring the egg donation to you. All you have to do is select an egg donor, freeze a semen sample, and sit back and relax.

In about forty-five to fifty days, the frozen embryos created with your semen and the donor eggs will arrive at your clinic. This process is successful because we use a fresh egg donation cycle and then freeze the resulting embryos.

We also guarantee a minimum of four blastocysts based on twelve to sixteen mature eggs per donor cycle. This approach has produced a number of amazing benefits that we never imagined when we started, and it seems to be the standard way of doing egg donation for the foreseeable future.

The benefits of doing egg donation using frozen embryos include:

- lower cost of treatment (you don't need to travel abroad),
- no travel fatigue (you can do the embryo transfer at your home clinic),
- no travel anxiety (you don't need to make a big trip to get treatment),
- less use of medication, or even your natural cycle (both
- have been shown to increase pregnancy success rates),
- perfect embryo transfer timing (your lab can thaw the embryos at a day's notice, so they can be transferred when the window of implantation is perfect, thereby increasing the success rate),
- no surprises with fertilization (you will know the results of the egg donation cycle well ahead),
- the ability to guarantee an outcome (we guarantee a minimum of four blastocysts, which brings you more than 50 percent closer to achieving an ongoing pregnancy),
- the same or better pregnancy rates than with fresh egg donation cycles,
- convenience for you (no travel, choose the time of treatment, no pressure),

- safety, familiarity and convenience of being treated at your home clinic.

This frozen embryo program is delivering the same or better pregnancy success rates than our fresh egg donation program. Everything is predictable and manageable. There is a set timeline for the delivery of embryos, the outcome is guaranteed, and your home clinic does not have to stress, since it knows it will be getting frozen embryos whose quality is easy to ascertain and measure.

Learn from the Experience of Others

If you are seeking egg donation, it is useful to learn from the experience of others who have gone before you. Some of the challenges that we have observed in our patients are acceptance and the grieving process, settling on an egg donor match, and keeping a high priority on getting on with life and having a child.

Acceptance is about agreeing to accept the concept that you need egg donation in order to successfully achieve an ongoing pregnancy and a child. If you are part of a couple, it's about being united in that decision. Realizing that you have no choice but to use an egg donor or semen donor is often accompanied by a multitude of emotions. "I never planned for this" is one of the first reactions, followed by anger, frustration, and other negative feelings. Those feelings are perfectly normal and to be expected. Everyone faced with this situation tends to go through a similar exasperation and grieving process.

Donor Matching is the process of identifying and accepting a donor match or even knowing what to look for in a donor. As time went on, we noticed an interesting phenomenon: most patients would appreciate seeing an egg donor who closely resembled them. However, even when the match was perfect, in 50 percent of the cases the newborn child did not have a resemblance to the intended mother, no matter how close the donor match. This was obviously due to the effect of the semen source, but it can also be observed in natural conception cases; the child has a good chance of not resembling the biological mother. The opposite was true as well. A donor, who was not necessarily a close match in appearance to the intended mother, resulted in an egg donation and a child who actually resembled the parents.

As third-party observers, we concluded that the results were too unpredictable either way, and impossible to control, and that the effort to reach a perfect match with the donor should be given lower importance than it was. Often the effort, and sometimes the agony, that you undergo in your pursuit of a look-alike does not result in the outcome you desire. We recommend you apply the 80/20 rule, whereby if the match is 80 percent in the direction you favor, then go along with that.

It would give you quicker time to treatment, reduced stress levels, and greater donor choice. In short, take a more flexible approach when you go through the donor selection process and make it easier on yourself to proceed into treatment. Everyone involved in the process has a limited capacity to control the outcome; in spite of the great technology, we are still at the mercy of nature and the universe's plan for our destiny. Patients who have taken this approach seem to have done better in treatment outcomes overall. They were more "go with the flow" types and while not everyone is born that way, releasing the reins a little during the donor matching process, and coming in with an open mind and flexibility, seems to reward patients.

Giving the treatment high priority. Over the years, I have met thousands of intended parents, but the behavior of a good number of them has amazed me. After all the investment and effort they placed on achieving a pregnancy, when it came down to the actual treatment, one or both of them would be flying around the world for business meetings. Or, a recipient mother would be exerting herself right after an embryo transfer as if the ordeal had never really happened, and jeopardizing the entire treatment and investment. My advice is to slow down around the treatment time. Relax and try to soak in the experience, giving your body and mind an opportunity to accept and connect with the embryos that will be transferred.

Egg donation may seem intimidating, strange, or unnatural at first. But, I am confident that if you are considering your options given a fertility challenge, you will realize that egg donation is a reasonable, kind, fair method of building a family, even though you may never have planned on it.

Amazing things can and usually do happen when you least expect them.

Surrogacy

For some intended parents, "gestational surrogacy" with or without egg donation, may be the only way to achieve a successful pregnancy. Gestational means that the surrogate mother, the "gestational carrier," is only agreeing to be implanted with your embryos (whether created from egg donation or with your eggs) in the IVF procedure. She does not donate her own eggs. This makes it a lot safer and easier for everyone involved because there is less emotional and biological connection between the surrogate and you.

Your legal rights are easy to protect and provide for, too. In "traditional surrogacy," the surrogate would be both the egg donor and the gestational carrier. You should avoid traditional surrogacy arrangements even if the cost seems lower than alternative options. The legal, biological, and emotional risks are just not worth it.

If you thought egg donation was daunting, surrogacy makes that look like child's play (no pun intended). Surrogacy arrangements are more akin to "surrogacy projects" and have many variables that need to be controlled. You should definitely seek the help of a professional, experienced agency to project manage your surrogacy journey, including the identification and recruitment of a surrogate, screening and legal coordination, medical coordination, and the logistics of the actual IVF cycle. Too many things need to be managed, and an agency plays a critical role in bringing everything together for you, the IVF clinic, lawyers, and surrogates.

Surrogacy can be used for challenges with the uterus of the intended mother, the absence of a uterus, an allergic reaction to medication used in IVF treatment, cancer treatment survivors, single intended fathers who do not have a female partner, or male gay couples who need a surrogate combined with egg donation. One important trend in surrogacy these days is the avoidance of transferring two or more embryos to the surrogate. Gay male couples especially, prefer to have at least two embryos transferred to the uterus of their surrogate, ideally one from each biological father. This allows them to complete their family in one surrogacy swoop, instead of doing surrogacy twice with a single child each time. We have successfully done the twin pregnancy approach for years, but this practice is now frowned upon by the medical community, especially in Canada, and we are changing with the times.

Best practices in the field of IVF today recommend the transfer of only one embryo at the blastocyst stage, especially when conceived from egg donation. This is particularly relevant to gay couples who, by default, use egg donation for the creation of their embryos when undergoing surrogacy. The same rule would apply to heterosexual couples. However, there is a chance that they would be allowed to transfer more than one embryo to their surrogate because the quality of their embryos could be relatively inferior to that of their gay counterparts, who would be using donor eggs. With donor eggs, the chance of high-quality embryos is greater, and therefore the probability of seeing a twin pregnancy is higher, by as much as 35 percent. The trend, therefore, is to avoid placing the burden of achieving a twin pregnancy on the surrogate. The other reason cited by the medical community is the avoidance of early delivery, which is closely associated with a twin pregnancy. Early delivery has also been linked to birth defects in one or both of the newborns, often resulting in greater intensive care costs for hospitals, government, or parents.

We currently offer surrogacy solutions in the USA, Canada, and Mexico. We felt options in other countries were too unstable legally, or inadequate medically to meet our high standards. The USA offers the most expensive route, albeit a convenient one. Canada is a great alternative to the USA and is less expensive, but suffers from long waiting lines for surrogates and little choice in surrogate selection.

Mexico is about half the cost of the USA and has a great supply of surrogates, although you have to be comfortable with the fact that communication with the surrogate will be more limited unless your command of Spanish is good.

All else being equal, Mexico is the most cost-effective and expedient choice. Ultimately, the process of surrogacy from a legal perspective is the same, regardless of the region you choose. The important thing to remember is that it takes time to organize—from four to six months—so the sooner you start your surrogate search, the better!

Chapter 8: Adoption

Waiting for Him

I have this list of my favorite baby names carefully tucked away in my day planner—a list that is eighty-four baby names long and eight years old. Every time I liked a name during the past eight years, I would pull out this list and scribble it down. Some were scratched off because a friend chose that name for her baby (or second or even third baby). Some have nicknames written beside them, or short forms we would use.

I love this list; it was always my reminder, my comfort, that someday I would become a mommy. Like many adoptive parents, we started with fertility treatments: cycle monitoring, IUI, donor sperm, donor embryos, IVF, ICSI, PESA, acupuncture, massage, yoga, herbs and vitamins. For years my world was my menstrual cycle, yet with every negative pregnancy test, I was not surprised. I can't explain why, but I could never really picture myself pregnant. I know this sounds ridiculous, especially when I think about how much we spent (financially and emotionally) on treatments. Every fiber of my being longed to be a mom, yet every negative pregnancy test just felt …right. And now when I look at my beautiful two-month-old son, I know why.

After our last treatment, which was really hard on me, my husband said that he just couldn't see me go through another cycle. Staring at that last negative pregnancy test he asked, "Why don't we look into adoption?" It was like a light bulb went off, and the whole world stood still. This was it; this was the reason I could never get pregnant.

Our Adoption Journey

All we knew about the adoption process was what we saw on television and in the movies, so we thought this would be easy compared to fertility treatments. I immediately went from full-time fertility patient to full-time adoption researcher, reading books, blogs, and articles and joining adoption support groups. I almost felt addicted to this new-found hope. Reading everything I could calmed my anxious (and impatient) nerves, but it quickly became overwhelming.

International, public, or private domestic adoption? What age range were we looking for? How long were we willing to wait? How comfortable were we not knowing the health history of the birth family? Open or closed adoption?

International Adoption

We were drawn to international adoption because it was top of mind, probably because it gets the most media attention (Angelina Jolie, Sandra Bullock, Modern Family). We also thought we wanted a closed adoption and international adoption would guarantee that. Our reasons had to do with our own interests—something that we eventually realized was not necessarily in the best interest of our future child.

I began researching international adoption specifically, and the intricacies of parenting a child of another race. I was feeling very confident and excited that we could do this! But there were very few options. Many countries were closing their programs or had long wait times. We weren't even eligible to adopt from many countries due to not being married long enough, or because my husband was approaching forty years of age. Many programs even had criteria for body weight! Every country had its own set of rules and there was no consistency. I was becoming increasingly frustrated. After looking into every program available, we finally decided to consider adopting from Bulgaria. The wait time was just less than three years for a child under three, the age restriction was liberal, and they didn't have any marriage-length criteria. We were pumped and so excited! We told our friends and family and they were all so thrilled and supportive.

We had a great discussion with the director of the program about how to get our dossier ready. We saw some pictures of the orphanages and were told some wonderful stories about successful adoptions and thrilled adoptive parents. Yet walking out of the room that day, something didn't feel right.

My husband noticed that the date on the photos was 1996. We felt uneasy and decided to think more about it. During the weeks ahead, we heard many horror stories about certain countries closing their programs randomly or leaving waiting couples hanging after they had paid a large deposit. Some families met their children but couldn't bring them home because a program closed unexpectedly.

We didn't have the stomach for that, so we had to think of something else.

Public Adoption

We considered adopting a child from foster care, but our local Children's Aid Society (CAS) told us that it would be at least a couple of years until our file would be looked at. The wait for an infant (a child under three in the public adoption world) could take up to eight years. We became incredibly deflated.

There is nothing like being told to "be patient" by a perfect stranger when you have been trying to become a mother for what feels like a thousand years. There was nothing about this process that we could control.

At our intake session, we were asked tough questions. Could we parent a child with fetal alcohol spectrum disorder (FASD) or autism, or one who had been exposed to trauma, neglect, or domestic violence? Things started to get real and the romance of adoption (what you see in the movies) started to transform. How many siblings could we handle? Would we consider adopting an older child?

My husband and I took a couple of days to answer those questions—ones you never expect to ask of yourself or your partner when starting a family. With public adoption, it's not about finding the perfect child for a family (what I thought when we started this journey), it's about finding the right families for these vulnerable children. It makes sense, but living this reality as a waiting adoptive parent is truly a challenge. It feels lonely.

Our CAS file was opened in September 2013. We were not contacted to be assigned a worker until September of 2015.

Meanwhile, our criteria changed from wanting a newborn to being open to a group of three siblings, up to seven years of age. It's amazing what time can do to a waiting adoptive parent. It can play games with your head and with your heart. During the longest two years of our lives, it was very difficult to stick to our comfort zone, but we had to remind ourselves what it was to avoid getting in over our heads.

Private Adoption and the Homestudy

While on the wait list at CAS we decided to pursue private domestic adoption. This could speed things up as a birth mother could potentially choose us right away. Like international adoption, the fees can get high but I didn't care. If it meant re-mortgaging our house, I was determined to make this happen.

When adopting, you must complete a homestudy (an assessment of your suitability as parents) and Parent Resources for Information, Development and Education (PRIDE) training. Overall, the process was a good experience, but it still felt unfair. We had to prove ourselves not only as parents, but as human beings after having already been put through the ringer of fertility treatments, which can make even the most self-assured person question their worth. Thankfully, we had a great worker who was compassionate and clicked with us right away.

Throughout the six-month home-study, we learned a lot about ourselves as individuals and as potential adoptive parents. We learned what it meant to have an open adoption and it became something we wanted. When our worker first spoke to us about it, we were completely closed to the idea. I feared that if the birth family was in our lives, then someday our child would choose them over us. It felt threatening. I wanted this child to be "ours" not "theirs." I had the naïve and wrong assumption that if the birth family wasn't around, it would be as if they didn't exist.

The more we learned about adoption from our own perspective, and through the eyes of our future child and their birth family, the more we realized that this could be the best thing. Our child would grow up knowing their roots, knowing they were loved, and not having those unanswered questions. They would grow up with some extra special family members who loved them as much as we did. It would be natural; it would be normal.

The Roller-Coaster Ride

In the beginning, my husband and I registered with three private agencies. Six months after completing our home study we were registered with six. There would have been more except a few never returned my calls. Some agencies were incredibly supportive, while others were happy to take our registration fee, never to be heard from again. Some let you know each time you are presented to a birth parent, while you have no idea if others even remember your name. It can start to feel like you are just another file in a drawer.

I was continuously updating our profile book and sending revisions in, hoping that changing a picture here or the wording there would make the difference and we would finally get chosen. This is what you do as waiting adoptive parents because if not, what else can you do? You wait. The waiting sometimes made my body ache. I could *feel* myself waiting.

While waiting for that phone call from an agency, it was very difficult to be present in my actual life. Waiting to adopt is ingrained in everything you do. When you are at the grocery store, you are waiting. When you are cooking dinner, you are waiting. When you are visiting family and friends, you are waiting. It's always there. Always in the back of your mind. It helped to take one day, even one *minute*, at a time.

We were presented to birth parents quite often, and each time was a roller-coaster ride of hope and disappointment. We were narrowed down to the "top two couples" several times.

Once we were even *interviewed* by birth parents because they could not decide between us and another couple. Our meeting went great and they told us she was expecting a baby girl. It was impossible not to let our minds run wild dreaming about tea parties and princesses. My husband is going to have a daughter. I am going to have a daughter.

Days passed and they still could not decide. After one full week of daydreaming and dread, we were told that the other couple was chosen instead of us. There was nothing to do except take a couple days and cry together.

"Just live your life and it will happen when you least expect it" were the words of wisdom we heard often from our well-meaning, loving friends and family. I am very goal-oriented. I was raised to think that when you worked hard for something it could happen and *would* happen. With adoption, it didn't matter how many agencies we registered with (six), how many profile book revisions we did (probably fifteen), or how many adoption websites we joined (three, not including the one I did myself). It didn't happen any faster and the whole thing sometimes felt like slow torture. Adoption is funny that way.

A couple of months later we were finally chosen by an expectant mother to adopt her baby girl! It was going to be an open adoption and we thought we had an amazing connection with this woman and her family. We studied my list of baby names together and decided on one that we all loved. It was perfect. She was perfect. Eight days after she was born, the birth mother changed her mind and decided to parent after all. No words come close to describing how we felt. We had to take a break, to shut out everything adoption. No agencies, no presentations, no blogs, books, or websites. We had to live—if only for a couple of months.

Eventually I started visualizing our life without kids. I would think about all the good things (my health, my loving husband, my great relationship with my family). I had to keep telling myself that life could be worse—much worse—although some days it didn't feel that way. It felt as though if one more person told me to be patient I would break down and cry. If anyone else said, "Everything happens for a reason" I would spontaneously combust.

I started to feel guilty for wanting something that would come from someone else's loss. It felt strange to want something so badly that in order for it to happen, another person would have to go through pain, grief, or even a crisis. A crisis separate yet parallel to my own. Adoption is as excruciating as it is beautiful. It is love and it is loss. As much as I resisted it, I eventually started to think that things do unfold as they should. I had to accept that there was a reason for all of this and we were exactly where we should be. People come into your life for a very special and specific reason.

For us, that very special and specific reason came almost exactly two years after we started our homestudy. We were chosen by an incredible young woman to be parents to her baby boy. Our love. Our *life*. It all makes sense now. We were waiting for him. He is perfect in every way. It's amazing our son even looks like us! There is no doubt in my mind that he was always meant to be ours. We absolutely love his birth family. They are *our* family. Our relationship with them just two months after he was born already feels natural and normal—as though it was supposed to happen. I am not sure why we had to go through so much pain to get what comes so easily to most people, but it doesn't matter now. Maybe it was to teach me a lesson in patience and gratitude. To stop trying to control what I can't control. I am sure that if having a child had come easily to us we would have loved him or her just the same-but something about this journey has humbled us completely. And you will never hear me complain about a midnight feeding!

Adoption as an Option to Grow Your Family: Demystifying the Process;

by Sofie Stergianis, MSW

So, you're thinking about adoption. In your mind you may be saying, "Just as I was beginning to understand the 'fertility treatment world,' now I have to learn about yet another option!"

A sense of self-doubt may come over you: "I failed at being a fertile person, and now I have to start the onerous task of adoption. I have to be *scrutinized,* and I may not pass." Let's demystify this process, so that by understanding it, you will come to realize that adoption is another very real and viable option to grow your family.

As an adoption professional, working in the field for almost forty years, I have worked with a multitude of families who have happily created or added to their families through adoption. On a personal level, after five years of unsuccessful fertility treatments (countless IUIs, five IVFs) and a miscarriage, I came to the point where I said "enough." Every adoptive family I have worked with has said to me about their child, "Everything I went through was for a reason, because I can't imagine parenting any other child than this one." That is how I feel about our son. Those five years of emotional and physical "torture" led us to *him*.

There is a path in adoption that will ultimately lead you to the child that you will parent. Let's look at the types of adoptions, the process, and then at the feelings you may expect to experience as you embark on choosing this path.

Types of Adoptions

There will be legislation where you live that outlines how adoption is governed, to make sure that everything is done ethically. Rules vary in different countries and jurisdictions, such as the United States, England, and Australia.[184] For a listing of all central authorities, worldwide, refer to the Hague website.[185]

Typically, there are three types of adoptions, and all three options can be explored simultaneously to build your family.

(1) Public Adoption

In a public adoption, the child is in the care of the child welfare system as a ward of the state. The child has either been removed from their home or relinquished by their birth family, and is living in a foster home. Available children range in age, with the most typical ages being toddlers to teenagers. There are no fees associated with a public adoption. You would apply to your local Children's Aid Society (CAS)[186] to start the process. Or, you can complete the paperwork privately, and then apply to the public system. In Ontario, there are a number of ways to access and apply for the "waiting children," including registering with your local CAS, going to the twice-yearly Adoption Resources Exchange (ARE)[187], where many Children's Aid Societies across the province present waiting children, and registering with

AdoptOntario[188], a databank of children legally free for adoption throughout the province.

(2) Private Adoption (known in some countries as Independent Adoption)

In a private adoption, a child's biological family makes the decision to pursue an adoption plan for their child, typically at birth, although the adoption option can be chosen at any age. The adoption is facilitated by a licensed adoption agency or individual licensee[189] on a fee-for-service basis. For several reasons, there are now far fewer adoptions of this type. The process involves a birth parent choosing adoptive applicants after looking at profiles created by the applicants.

Many people say that this profile is like a "marketing piece," but birth parents do not look at these profiles to choose a family with the best house or car. They choose based on a connection that they feel. For example, one of the reasons our son's birth mother chose us was because we had a large extended family, and she had no family. This was important to her, to have her birth son enveloped in love.

Once you are chosen, you typically meet the birth parent or possibly the birth family. Keep an open mind about meeting the birth family. Right now, you may be thinking, "I just want a child, I don't want to adopt the entire family." Understanding the importance of the birth family in your lives is something that develops and grows. Ultimately, many people choose an open adoption, even though initially they might have been afraid of it, because it is in the best interest of their child—no secrecy or shame. The birth family becomes a natural part of your entire extended family constellation. As my son said when he was, after being asked how he felt about visiting with his birth family, "Of course I want to visit Mom. You have your side of the family, dad has his side of the family, and I have my side of the family. And we are all one big family, right Mom?" From the mouths of babes, this is what open adoption is.

Every jurisdiction has laws related to birth parent signing of adoption consents, and rights in terms of revoking their consents after the placement. In Ontario, birth parents cannot sign adoption consents until seven days after the baby is born. Whatever day they do end up signing, they then have twenty-one days to change their minds. This period is the most difficult, and if you know in your heart that you would not be able to "survive" a birth parent changing their mind and the baby going back to them, then you would not choose this kind of adoption. You would look at the public or international adoption route.

(3) Inter-Country Adoption (or International Adoption)

Inter-country adoption involves the adoption of a child from another country, with the children living in orphanages, baby homes, or some other form of state care, or living with a relative if it is a relative adoption. In Ontario, inter-country adoption must be facilitated through a licensed adoption agency that is authorized to facilitate adoption by the Ministry of Children, Community and Social Services[190] and the child's country of origin. Services are provided on a fee-for-service basis and vary depending on the adoption agency's fee schedule. The agency is responsible for preparing the dossier for the foreign authority, including translation, notarization, and authentication of the documents. They are responsible for presenting you with a child proposal that includes all of the medical and social history information.

If the country you live in has signed the Hague Convention on Protection of Children and Co-operation in Respect of Inter-country Adoption (the Hague Convention), they must follow the rules and process as set out in the Hague Convention.

The Hague Convention[191] "protects children and their families against the risks of illegal, irregular, premature or ill-prepared adoptions abroad. … It also seeks to prevent the abduction, the sale of, or traffic in children."

The Adoption Process

Homestudy

In order to adopt, the main requirement is completing a homestudy. You may be thinking, "They are going to judge me based on my home?" A homestudy is not a study of your home. It is an assessment of you as adoptive applicants. People say that it is unfair that anyone who can have a child by birth does not need to be assessed, and yet adoptive families do. However, the assessment is not to see if you are "perfect" people. In fact, adoption practitioners always talk about how "survivors make great parents." If you have "survived" a challenging life situation, or a loss, and have grown from this experience, this is a strength.

The assessment, in fact, is based on your readiness to adopt and your understanding of adoption as applicants.

Let's talk first about your "readiness to adopt." Part of the psychological component of adopting is that you will probably feel unsure about your decision, right up to when they are placing the child in your arms. This is not like giving birth where even if you have reservations, the child is arriving.

In this process, it is all about logical thinking. You meet with professionals, are asked intrusive questions, fill out paperwork, are fingerprinted—none of this feels like what it should in terms of creating a family. At any point, you can step back and say, "This is too much for me. This does not feel good." And you probably will. This is what I call "the adoption dance," forwards and backwards. This is so normal, and does not mean that adoption is not the right decision. It means your brain is processing something that is outside your comfort zone.

Typically, in a couple's adoption process, there is the "dragger" and the "draggie." One of the two in a couple usually gets to the decision of adopting faster than the other one. If you are the "draggie" in this adoption process, everything might feel daunting and unnatural, and you can't possibly imagine having a family out of this artificial process. As a "dragger," you feel badly that you are always pushing, and possibly arguing, about a direction that you know is the right one, even though sometimes you even doubt it. That is why a home-study is so important. To discuss these feelings, to process your reservations, and to learn more about why you are responding the way you are.

The home-study is an assessment, but equally importantly, it has a learning component. Coming to understand how parenting by birth is different from parenting through adoption is the goal. The day-to-day parenting is the same for the most part, but adoptive parents have an added responsibility that biological parents do not: to raise their child to develop an honest understanding of their adoption, and to assist their child in developing a healthy self-esteem as an adopted person. So when at age nine my son realized that he would never have birth father history, he looked at me with sadness and pain in his eyes, and said, "Do you know what it's like Mom, not knowing what half of you is? Not knowing who you look like, where your talents come from, what your nationality is … Do you know what it's like Mom?" All I could say was, "No. Tell me what it's like for you." My job as an adoptive parent is to help my son grieve his loss, and to feel good about himself, regardless.

Here are some other examples of learning, to help you understand how parenting by birth is different from parenting through adoption. A family who adopted a five-year-old called me a week later, ecstatic that their daughter had bonded so well with them, always hugging them and going to them.

Then they called a few days later, upset, as they had found that she was just as affectionate with the neighbors, whom she did not know, and was ready to go home with them. This is indiscriminate attachment, and when children are first placed it may occur. This is what adoptive families need to understand and learn to address. Then there was the family who adopted a four-month-old baby internationally. You may think, "Four months old, the adjustment will be easy." But this child had only ever been with his foster mother. When he left her to come to Canada, he was in shock. For the first six months, all he did was sleep and stare out with a blank gaze. His parents thought something was very wrong with him. Then one day he woke up and he was a different little boy. "It was like the light went on," his parents stated; he had attached. It is this kind of learning, and all the learning necessary to help your child as they grow with their healthy identity, that is addressed during the homestudy process.

In Ontario, the format used to complete a homestudy is called Structured Analysis, Family Evaluation (SAFE). This format is used for private, inter-country, and public adoption, and is portable across all three systems. The homestudy involves a series of interviews, and supporting documents are also required, which normally include, but are not limited to, police clearances, medical reports, child welfare checks, and references. To complete a homestudy, you either have to use a CAS adoption worker or a ministry-approved private adoption practitioner. If you are using a private adoption practitioner, you choose whom to work with. It is so important to feel a connection with this person, as they will guide you to make very important decisions. You can find a list of private adoption practitioners in Ontario at the Ministry of Children, Community and Social Services.[192] The homestudy typically takes four to six months to complete and is valid for two years, at which time you need an update to document any changes. This will involve obtaining new references, criminal and child welfare clearances, and medical reports, and meeting with an adoption professional to update your information.

In some provinces, states, or countries, a mandatory training course is a prerequisite for completing the homestudy assessment. In Ontario, the training required is called PRIDE (Parent Resources for Information, Development and Education) pre-training. It is a twenty-seven-hour training program, and is divided into nine modules. The curriculum includes such topics as attachment; loss and grief; talking about adoption with the child; the effects of neglect, lack of stimulation, abuse, and institutionalization on children; open adoption; identity formation and the importance of cultural and racial awareness, etc.

As a PRIDE trainer, I see people walk in the door on the first day with the look, "Why do I have to do this?" At the end of the training, they leave feeling empowered, having learned so much, stating that they can't imagine adopting without this training program. The Ontario Association of Children's Aid Societies (OACAS) is the license holder of PRIDE pre-service in Ontario, and you can either complete the training via a CAS at no cost, or with a private PRIDE trainer for a fee. You can find a schedule of private PRIDE training sessions at the AdoptOntario[193] website.

The extent of information you get about the child you hope to adopt depends on the type of adoption you pursue. A child proposal includes social and medical information—sometimes there is a great deal of information, sometimes there is limited information. When exploring what route will be best for you, many factors will be taken into consideration: costs, time frames, age and health of children, requirements of each system or country of the adoptive parents, etc. This is what you will learn during the homestudy process and the training, so that you can make a decision based on what makes sense for you and your family. Talking to agencies, other adoptive families, your adoption practitioner—all this will lead you to the adoption "path" where your child is waiting.

Completing all of the requirements for adoption takes some time, and this time depends on the system you choose to pursue. For example, in Ontario your local CAS may have a waiting list for the PRIDE training or to complete your homestudy because of limited staffing or resources. Working with a private adoption practitioner is usually a faster process, as it is fee-for-service, so you can decide whom to work with based on your desired time frames. In all three systems, children are placed based on the match with the family. How long the matching will take, and the subsequent placement of a child, depends on the type of adoption you are pursuing and the profile of the child you are hoping to adopt. Is it a roller-coaster ride, as the mom discovers in, "Waiting for Him" elsewhere in this chapter? Yes, it can be. But if you hang on tight, you will make it through the ups and downs.

Each province in Canada has its own adoption laws, regulations, policies, and procedures that must be followed. If you reside outside of Ontario, contact your provincial Central Adoption Authority11 to get further information. You must follow the adoption protocol of your province to complete a homestudy and any education requirements to obtain provincial approval to adopt.

Positive Adoption Language

As you explore adoption, you might want to be aware of your "language" in this area. By using positive adoption language, we are reinforcing the idea that adoption is not second best, just a different way to create a family. When people ask, "Do you have any children of your *own*?" or, "Do you know anything about the *real* parents?" the implication is that the child is not your own and that you are not a real family. We don't question whether two people who are not related by blood are members of the same family; you and your spouse, you and your in-laws, you are family. But people question the relationship in adoption, even though you are linked by law and by love.

So be careful of saying, "We decided to adopt because we could not have a child *of our own*." You are already setting things up for your family and friends to feel that this child is not "yours." That word own is very powerful. Imagine your child at age five hearing, "We could not have a child *of our own* so we decided to adopt." "Mom, Dad, I'm not your own?"

It is better to say, "We could not have a child by birth." Start practicing these words now so that when someone asks about the "real" parents, you will always reply, "Do you mean the birth parents?" What you answer after that, you will get more direction on through the adoption process. This is what you're learning will be during the homestudy and the PRIDE training.

The Psychology of Adoption

The most difficult aspect of making the leap to adopt after infertility is acknowledging that we don't always get what we want in life. Recognize that adoption is another choice, not a failure. Adoption may not have been your *first* choice, but it became your choice. You could have chosen to remain child free, or not had another child, for those with secondary infertility. Deciding that you *really* wanted to add a child to your family unit was ultimately what you chose.

Acknowledging that this is not how you *thought* you were going to create your family, and feeling comfortable grieving this as a loss that will be with you forever, is important. There is a mythology that we have to be "resolved" in our infertility grief before we move on to adoption. There might always be a tiny part of you that will always grieve the birth child you did not have. This does not mean that you do not love the child you adopt. You can love your child, and still grieve the child you did not give birth to. Those two things are separate.

Something may come up through the years that reminds you of this loss. That could be when your family is sitting at the dinner table, talking about how much your sibling's new child looks exactly like them. Or, when you wonder if your in-laws will love your child who joined the family through adoption as much as they love the new biological grandchild. You will come to the point where you acknowledge any feelings of loss that come up, tuck them back in, and move on. Just as your child can grieve the fact that their birth parent "gave them up," and still love you as their parent.

The psychology of adoption involves understanding and accepting that every adoption begins with loss. The joys of adoption are clear and quite profound. But all the studies show that unless you understand the losses, you cannot have a healthy adoption. The child loses the opportunity to grow up in their birth family and possibly their culture, the birth parents lose the opportunity to parent their child, and you lose the opportunity to have this child as your birth child.

Let's do a little exercise to help you with thinking about these losses. Do it with your partner if you are in a coupled relationship. Take a piece of paper, and write the following:

What are the losses for *you*, not having *this* child (your adopted child) as a birth child, even if you have children by birth. Write down as many as you can think of, until you have exhausted every single one. For example, one of the losses might be that the child will not inherit your sense of humor, although having a birth child does not guarantee that the child would either (they could have your mother-in-law's dry sense of humor). Or the loss may be that you did not experience a pregnancy. After you have written them all down, look at them, feel sad, and know that it is OK to feel sad. Only then can you move on to love the child that does come into your home.

Let's do one last short exercise. On a piece of paper, each of you write down what you think your "fantasy child" would be—what the child looks like, what his/her personality is like.

Take time to write down everything that you can think of. Are you done? Now that you have completed this, take the piece of paper and hide it. This child may never become real for you, and the child you do end up adopting may be nothing like your fantasy child—just as your birth child may have been nothing like your fantasy child. Unless you let this fantasy child go, you cannot love the child that comes to you through adoption.

This is an area to work on through the adoption process, something you should feel comfortable to speak about with your adoption practitioner or an independent therapist. My professional and personal experience in adoption has led me to truly understand that "Life is not in absolutes!" We change our direction in life because we have to, and we then often realize that this is where we were meant to be.

Making the successful leap from infertility to adoption entails a willingness to look at adoption and say, "This is a good way to make a family." Acknowledge the journey, that you are not where you thought you would be, but that each step opens new doors and an incredible new path. Don't be afraid to venture onto this new path. I am forever grateful that my five years of fertility treatments, pain, and great sadness led me to the child I adore, and I truly feel I was meant to parent.

I am not alone in this thought as an adoptive parent, and have heard this repeatedly from adoptive parents over the last three-and-a-half decades. I love the words that poet Jaime Frodyma wrote, "I did not give you the gift of life—life gave me the gift of you." My parting words to you then, as you contemplate adoption and wonder if you will be a "normal" family, are these: We are not "different" families. Our families were formed in a different way.

Acknowledgments:

A warm thank you to two special friends and colleagues for your insights and contributions. Thank you to Sharon Gollert, MSW, RSW, AccFM and Jan Silverman MA, M.Ed. Most importantly, thank you to my son Adam, for teaching me more about adoption than any of the seminars I have been to, the books I have read, or the families I have worked with, because now I feel it in my heart. It is an absolute joy to be your mother.

---

[184] Adopt US Kids, (USA), http://www.adoptuskids.org/; Coram BAAF, (UK), http://corambaaf.org.uk; The Hague Convention, "Australia: Central Authority," https://www.hcch.net/en/states/authorities/details3/?aid=48.

[185] The Hague Convention, https://www.hcch.net/en/home.
[186] Ontario Association of Children's Aid Societies, www.oacas.org.
[187] Adoption Resource Exchange, http://www.children.gov.on.ca/htdocs/English/topics/adoption/how/conference.aspx.
[188] Ministry of Children, Community and Social Services, Ontario, "Adoptions Licensees," http://www.children.gov.on.ca/htdocs/English/adoption/decided-to-adopt/privatelicensees.aspx.
[189] Ministry of Children, Community and Social Services, Ontario, "Licensed International Adoption Agencies," http://www.children.gov.on.ca/htdocs/English/adoption/decided-to-adopt/internationaladoption.aspx
[190] The Hague Convention, "Adoption Section," https://www.hcch.net/en/instruments/conventions/specialised-sections/intercountry-adoption.
[191] Ministry of Children, Community and Social Services, Ontario, "Adoption Practitioners," http://www.children.gov.on.ca/htdocs/English/adoption/decided-to-adopt/practitioners.aspx
[192] AdoptOntario, "PRIDE," https://secure.adoptontario.ca/pride.main.aspx.
[193] Governement of Canada, Citizenship and Immigration, "Provincial and Territorial Central Adoption Authorities," https://www.canada.ca/en/immigration-refugees-citizenship/services/canadians/adopt-child-abroad/authorities.html

Chapter 9: Frequently Asked Questions

Naturopathic Medicine

Can Anti-Müllerian Hormone (AMH) levels (which is reflective of ovarian reserve) be improved?

AMH goes down each year and generally doesn't go up. It may improve, but don't make this your goal or focus. Many people think that AMH represents a woman's egg quality, but it is merely a number that reflects her ovary reserve. It tells us if you have a lot of follicles or very few follicles remaining in your ovaries ready to ovulate and potentially create babies.

This blood test can be used as a tool to understand how your ovaries may respond under a medicated stimulation prior to IVF. On its own, AMH is not a predictive tool to assess your ability to conceive or achieve a healthy pregnancy outcome. You may have a high AMH in the case of Polycystic Ovary Syndrome (PCOS) and you may have a very low AMH in the case of premature ovary insufficiency (POI). In the case of a woman with PCOS and a high AMH, she may be a good candidate for IVF and in the case of a woman with POI and extremely low AMH she is less likely to be a good candidate for IVF. Changing your AMH levels (even in these two latter extreme cases) won't improve your fertility since the AMH level would only change marginally. The goal ultimately, is to ensure you are regularly ovulating healthy eggs and changing the AMH won't affect your outcome.

Do anti-oxidants really work to improve egg quality and sperm quality?

Yes, anti-oxidants from eating fruits and vegetables improve egg quality and sperm quality but bigger and better studies are needed to find appropriate dosing of the various anti-oxidants in supplement. There is a very important and delicate balance between the levels of Reactive Oxygen species (ROS) and anti-oxidant levels found naturally in the follicular fluid surrounding the ova of a follicle and in men's semen. ROS are formed as a natural by-product of the normal metabolism of oxygen and have important roles in cell signalling and homeostasis. If ROS levels are too high and this imbalance is disturbed by inflammatory processes created by certain offending agents such as cigarette smoke, a low nutrient dense diet, stress, conditions such as PCOS and endometriosis, then significant damage to cell structures occur, egg quality is affected and women endure subfertility.

This is where anti-oxidants through healthy nutrition choices and supplementation may help because they can re-balance the ROS-anti-oxidant ratio in both a man's semen and woman's follicles.

What's the best diet for fertility?

It really depends on the cause of your subfertility and whether or not you need to lose weight since a healthier Body Mass Index (BMI) improves your chances of pregnancy and live birth outcome. The medical literature has often quoted the Mediterranean diet as the best diet for chronic illness prevention, healthy aging and for fertility. The Mediterranean diet consists of vegetables, fruits, potatoes, legumes, whole grains, dairy, red meat, fish, poultry, olive oil, and a little alcohol. There was a study done in 2019 in "The American Journal of Obstetrics and Gynecology on the best diet for fertility called "Dietary Patterns and Outcomes of assisted reproduction" and they found that the higher the adherence to the Mediterranean diet the better the pregnancy and live birth outcome. They also observed an even better outcome with the following modifications to the Mediterranean diet that they called the "pro-fertility diet"; which includes higher intake of supplemental folic acid, vitamin B12, vitamin D, low-pesticide fruits and vegetables, whole grains, seafood, dairy, and soy foods, and a lower intake of high-pesticide fruits and vegetables. This "pro-fertility diet" had higher odds of live birth by up to 50%. Remember though that you should be treated as an individual and diet modified based on your individual condition, nutrient deficiencies, food sensitives and personal needs.

In order to improve my fertility do I really need to be 100% strict with healthy eating?

No. Do your best. However, the mere fact that you suffer from infertility means you likely inherited a condition that carries with it a predisposition to an imbalanced ROS-Antioxidant ratio. This means that you do need to eat healthier than the average person in order to improve your egg quality or sperm quality. There should be some flexibility, since over focusing on healthy eating can be a stress in and of itself. Eating perfectly is a challenging concept in a world full of endless unhealthy food choices especially since a large portion of the population eats very poorly and they still conceive without issues. However, also do your best to change your perception when you make healthy food choices. Think of healthy nutrition in terms of abundance instead of using a scarcity mentality.

Remind yourself that you are not being punished by being told you need to make healthy food choices and think of it as a way to expand your palate with the huge variety healthy foods that exist. Think of food as medicine. You may also consider you won two lotteries. The first lottery isn't an ideal one…the one that bestowed subfertility upon you. The second lottery is that your subfertility has acted as a red-flag to warn you that healthy changes are needed and by eating an anti-oxidant rich diet you are slowing down the entire body's aging process and improving the rest of your body while you treat the condition that is causing your subfertility. Without subfertility, maybe you wouldn't have gotten to know your body so well and recognized your body's need for healthier food choices.

If you eat healthier now and for the long term; you will be healthier as an individual and one day, ideally as a parent.

Acupuncture and East Asian Medicine

Can acupuncture help with male factor infertility?

Approximately 40-50% infertility cases are considered to be related to male factors.[194] However, acupuncture application to male infertility has not attracted much attention. Although traditionally, acupuncture has been used to treat various male reproductive health issues for many decades, the vast majority of infertility patients seen in many acupuncture clinics are women. There has been a limited amount of studies conducted on male infertility and acupuncture. However, some researchers have reported encouraging results. Clinical studies have shown that acupuncture may help patients with low sperm concentration[195], poor morphology,[196] [197] and low motility.[198] [199] A placebo-controlled study on patients with severe oligoasthenozoospermia (reduced sperm motility and count), published in *Fertility and Sterility*, concluded that patients who received acupuncture twice a week for six weeks significantly improved their sperm motility.[6] In some cases, herbal medicine, in conjunction with acupuncture, can be beneficial in treatment of male infertility. Series of studies in Japan showed that administrations of Kampo herbal formulas could be helpful in improving sperm concentration and motility.[200] The response to acupuncture or herbal medicine can vary depending on each individual case. As the sperm regeneration process takes about 64 days (ranging between 42 to 76 days),[201] a significant change in sperm analysis should not be expected within a short period of receiving acupuncture or herbal therapy. We usually recommend the trial treatment for a period of three months in order to determine the patient's response to the treatment.

Does acupuncture help women with diminished ovarian reserve?

We have frequently been seeing patients with diminished or low ovarian reserve issues. Lab results of those patients often show low antimüllerian hormone (AMH), low antral follicle count (AFC) and elevated baseline (cycle day 3) FSH level.

These numbers are essential for patients who are undergoing IVF as these parameters could predict their response to IVF medications. Although some reports suggested that acupuncture and moxibustion may help these biomarkers [202][203][204], the actual numbers in lab results do not always notably improve for some patients. However, it is important to note that the diminished ovarian reserve does not mean you cannot get pregnant. Also, it does not necessarily indicate that you have a lesser chance when attempting to conceive naturally. In a paper published in the Journal of American Medical Association in 2017, the researcher concluded that women of advanced reproductive age with biomarkers of diminished ovarian reserve (low AMH or high FSH) were not associated with reduced fecundability or a lower cumulative probability of conceiving naturally.[205] Their study somewhat confirmed my clinical observations. It explained cases that sometimes surprised me. Over the years, I have seen quite a few patients with a diminished ovarian reserve who spontaneously became pregnant while having acupuncture and moxibustion. Some of them successfully conceived and carried to term more than once. Similar cases are also reported by other acupuncturists.[206] Please note that remarkable success does not happen to every patient. However, I wanted to share our experience, as I have encountered many patients visit our clinic who were devastated upon hearing the news about their poor ovarian reserve. There is always hope.

Mind-Body Awareness

Do any of these actual comments resonate with you, or apply to your situation, and if not, which other ones come to mind?

- "I feel pressured for time, it's running out!"
- "I can't keep on living this way, I'm depressed."
- "Every time we have sex it's painful."
- "Part of me feels that I can't keep my career and have a baby; I can't have both."
- "I have a hard time feeling relaxed."
- "If I have a baby, I'll lose my freedom."
- "We're in our 40's now and I feel pressed for time, I wanted it earlier and she put it off."

Some reasons that I've heard why people want a baby, and what thinking I believe contributes to blocking it:

- "To have someone to love and they'll love me back"
- "My husband is losing patience with me"
- "I feel there's obligation with family, especially my in-laws"
- "I don't want to be alone in my old age"
- "My wife wants it and I don't really care"
- "My husband works all the time and I'm lonely"
- "Our culture says we're supposed to have a baby after we marry"

Can you help us with our relationship because I feel we're missing the intimate connection? We haven't had a good foundation right from the beginning.

Absolutely, a good solid relationship is essential, it's your 'nest'.

My parents didn't like being parents; do you think that has anything to do with me sometimes feeling like I don't want to be a parent either?

Yes, it can. Lots of times as a child we make assumptions/jump to conclusions about what we see or hear the adults in our lives talking or arguing about, and it might be just that simple that you decided way back then to not go through that pain and be a parent like them.

Can you help me with performance anxiety because I feel like I need to perform to have a baby?

Yes. We'd need to discover how you truly feel inside – whether you really want a baby or not because sometimes we're not being honest with ourselves. For example, only saying yes to our partner in order to please them or wanting to have a child for the wrong reason.

"I believe most physical ailments are tied emotionally, caused from frightening unexpected events that are often the trigger that sets off illness and dis-ease, or block us from having what we want in life. When we uncover, resolve and release these, people heal themselves and return to wholeness." Glenda I Johnson

Counseling

How do you manage the mixed emotions when you're socializing with others who are pregnant or who have children?

Of course, it's really uncomfortable to have the sometimes-conflicting emotions when, on one hand, you're happy for other people's pregnancies or ability to have children, but on the other hand, you're sad that you've not yet been able to build your family. Some strategies that might help include:

1. Identify the emotions that you're feeling.
2. Try to put your own needs first before the needs of others. If you're not comfortable attending a social event, give yourself permission not to attend. If you're not sure if you want to attend the event, consider how to attend "in a safe way". For example, perhaps plan to go for just a short time, think who you feel comfortable talking to, and limit the conversation to only what you feel you're able to discuss.
3. Have a "script" prepared so that you're not caught off guard when others ask you intrusive questions (e.g., "When are you going to have children?")

My partner and I have been putting our lives on hold since trying to have a baby. We feel that life is passing us by. What can we do?

It's very understandable that you've been putting such effort in to having a baby, and you don't want to make decisions about other parts of your life that might need to be changed once you're pregnant. However, trying to have a child is like swimming across a pond. You've left one shore (i.e., you're going through the process of "trying"), but you've not yet reached the other shore (i.e., when you have your baby in your arms). Your job is to figure out how to stay afloat while you're still "swimming". It's important to continue to build your life and create joy and meaning in your life so that you have the resources to continue "trying" to have a child. It's also important to understand that, in "growing" your world and not putting your life on hold, if you need to make changes in your life once you have a child, you can do that. In the meantime, give yourself permission to enjoy your life even while trying to have a baby.

Medical Route to Conception

What are the side effects of fertility medications?

The important thing to realize is that most patients have minimal, if any side effects. Some women may experience hot flashes, emotional changes, bloating, headaches and nausea. These occur in about 5-10% of patients. The most common one we have to address is the risk of multiple pregnancy.

Naturally occurring rates for twins are 2%, while with fertility drugs this can increase to 10-20%. This is why monitoring the ovarian response while you are on fertility medications is so important, especially if you are having intercourse or doing an intrauterine insemination, where we cannot control how many embryos actually implant versus with in vitro fertilization, where we put in the number of embryos we hope will lead to a healthy pregnancy.

How effective are fertility treatments?

We have to put this into perspective in terms of our natural fertility. When we are in our twenties, our likelihood of getting pregnant is about 25% per month. As women get older, this number goes down to 10% by the time we are 38, and 5% by the time we are 40. The overall success rates for intrauterine inseminations with oral medications is about 10%, while with injectable medications it is about 20%. In vitro fertilization pregnancy rates can reach up to 70-80% in women under the age of 35, or with egg donation or preimplantation genetic screening, however, in women over the age of 40, the success rates with their own eggs are 10-20%. The other thing to remember is these are what we call "pregnancy rates", which do not take into account the possibility of miscarriage. Therefore, more recently, we have focused on talking about "live birth rates" or the likelihood of actually taking home a baby at the end of the treatment. These range from 55% under age 35, to about 4-12% over the age of 40.

Egg donation and Surrogacy

What do I need for starting the process of IVF treatment with an egg donor?

The first step is to fill out our online Find a Donor Form and inform us of your preferred criteria for a donor. Once completed, you will be assigned with a personal Donor Coordinator.

Your Coordinator will talk you through your options for egg donation and answer any questions you may have about the procedure. Once you fully understand our process and you have selected your egg donor, you will receive an agreement to sign. A deposit is also required to secure your egg donor.

We will then work together with your fertility clinic to begin your IVF treatment, while closely monitoring your progress. Our team will provide you with guidance during your journey and up until you achieve a pregnancy.

How many eggs (oocytes) should I expect to receive?

You will receive a minimum of 10 oocytes using ELITE IVF's fertility treatment, provided you are not sharing a donor with other recipients (through our shared fresh egg donor program). On average, we collect in the range of 12-16 oocytes from our egg donors. If there is any excess it is allocated to your treatment, along with the 12-16 eggs.

Is there an age limit for intended parents to be accepted into the egg donation program?

While your age is taken into account, the primary factors in determining if you are a good candidate for an egg donation depends on the physical examination of the medical team. Our specialist(s) will review your overall health, condition of your uterus and your ability to both sustain a pregnancy and deliver a baby after entering the egg donation program. Our specialist medical team will confirm your acceptance accordingly. Our egg donation program provides an opportunity to use oocytes of a person who has proven fertility, meaning there is a high probability of fertilization and implantation. ELITE IVF's intended parents typically range in age from late 20s to early 50s.

Adoption

Is age a factor in your eligibility to be accepted as an applicant for adoption?

The assessment is based on what is in the best interest of a child, and age can be a factor. Adoption agencies, private and international, as well as Children Aid Societies, have policies &/or best practice guidelines that speak to the age of an applicant, as well as the applicant in relation to the age of the child they will adopt. For example, some international countries have it written into their law what the maximum age difference should be between a child and a parent. In private domestic adoption, the birth parent/parents choose the adoptive parents, and age is just one factor in their decision. In all the different options to adopt, usually, the older you are, the older a child you will be considered for.

What is the "fastest" way to adopt?

When you are ready to move forward with your adoption plans, your adoption practitioner will guide you on how to research, and help you with your decision making as to which path you will choose to pursue. There will be many factors that your decision will be based on, including children's ages, culture, race, financial considerations, etc. You might choose one path to pursue, or, you might pursue multiple paths at the same time.

How much will adoption cost?

Adoption through the Child Welfare system is free, as it is a government service covered through your tax dollars. Not including the home study and any mandatory training programs, a private adoption is approximately between $25,000-$30,000, and after an initial retainer, the remaining fees are paid in stages. An international adoption is $25,000 and up, depending on the country, and the fees are paid over the waiting period.

How can we guarantee we get a healthy child?

No one can guarantee a healthy child, as genetically, they are no guarantees that your child will be healthy. You will receive information about the child and/or the birth family, to be able to make an informed decision about your comfort level in moving forward with the adoption.

---

[194] Kumar, N. et al., Trends of male factor infertility, an important cause of infertility: A review of literature. J Hum Reprod Sci. 2015 Oct-Dec; 8(4): 191-196.

[195] Siterman S, Eltes F, Wolfson V, Lederman H, Bartoov B. Does acupuncture treatment affect sperm density in males with very low sperm count? A pilot study. Andrologia 2000;32:31-9

[196] Gurfinkel E, Cedenho AP, Yamamura Y, Srougi M. Effects of acupuncture and moxa treatment in patients with semen abnormalities. Asian J Androl 2003;5:345-8.

[197] Pei J, Strehler E, Noss U, Abt M, Piomboni P, Baccetti B, Sterzik K. Quantitative evaluation of spermatozoa ultrastructure after acupuncture treatment for idiopathic male infertility. Fertil Steril 2005;84: 141-7.

[198] Siterman S, Eltes F, Wolfson V, Zabludovsky N, Bartoov B. Effect of acupuncture on sperm parameters of males suffering from subfertility related to low sperm quality. Arch Androl 1997;39:155-61.

[199] Dieterle, S., Li, C., Greb, R., Bartzsch, F., Hatzmann, W., Huang, D. A prospective randomized placebo-controlled study of the effect of acupuncture in infertile patients with severe oligoasthenozoospermia *Fertility and Sterility*, 2009 Oct;92(4):1340-3.

[200] Terasawa K, Kita T, Sekiya N. *Male Infertility*. EBM Kampo. 2nd ed. Tokyo: Ishiyaku Publishers; 2007.

[201] Misell, LM., et al., A stable isotope-mass spectrometric method for measuring human spermatogenesis kinetics in vivo. J Urol. 2006 Jan;175(1):242-6

[202] Zeng, Y. Effects of transcutaneous electrical acupoint stimulation on ovarian reserve of patients with diminished ovarian reserve in invitro fertilization and embryo transfer cycles. J Obstet Gynaecol Res. Volume41, Issue12 December 2015 Pages 1905-1911

[203] 2. Dong XL, Ran JK, Zhang HJ, Chen K, Li HX. [Acupuncture combined with medication improves endocrine hormone levels and ovarian reserve function in poor ovarian response patients undergoing in vitro fertilization-embryo transplantation]. Zhen ci yan jiu =*Acupuncture Research*. 2019 Aug;44(8):599-604.

[204] Zhen Jiu, Z. et al., [Effects of moxibustion at Shenshu (BL 23) on level of sex hormones and AMH in sub-health peri-menopausal women]. Zhongguo Zhen Jiu. 2017 Apr 12;37(4):381-385.

[205] Steiner, Z. et al. Association Between Biomarkers of Ovarian Reserve and Infertility Among Older Women of Reproductive Age JAMA. 2017;318(14):1367-1376

[206] Moon, Hyon-Ju. et al., A Case Report on Four Pregnancies of Subfertile Patients with Low Anti-Müllerian Hormone (AMH) Level after Korean Medical Treatments. J Korean Obstet Gynecol. 2015 VOL.28 NO.2 : 174-182

Closing

This book has been a dream of mine for many years now and I am so happy that it has finally come to fruition. From its inception and putting together all the different fertility resources, through to its completion, it has been a wonderful, humbling, learning and illuminating journey. While some things went very smoothly, other unexpected obstacles surfaced, very much akin to the roller coaster of emotions I felt during my fertility journey.

I have learned so much during this process, from what we can do with lifestyle interventions such as diet and exercise, to Eastern modalities like acupuncture and herbs, and mind-body practices like NLP and hypnosis. There are also the many facets of couples' counseling, medical treatments, the use of donor sperm and donor eggs, and gestational carriers; and the intricacies of adoption. And for some, there is living without realizing their dream of having children.

I am grateful to all my co-authors and to the patients who have been brave and kind enough to share their stories in the hopes of helping others. I am honored to have Dr. Rankin and Dr. Northrup endorse this project and cannot thank them enough for taking the time to review the manuscript.

I hope that by reading this book, you have found what you needed. Trying to become a parent can be one of life's hardest and most heartbreaking journeys. However, you are not alone. In sharing these resources with you, I hope you feel empowered to be, do, have and become whatever you need, so that you can endure your fertility journey with grace, as well as a deeper appreciation of how this particular challenge has helped you to grow and expand.

I often wonder why I fell in love with this field during my obstetrics and gynecology residency and why my application was accepted one day late. I've also wondered why I experienced the heartache of struggling to conceive. What brings me peace is knowing that there must have been a divine intervention that orchestrated my life in the most synchronistic way possible, so that I may share with others what I learned on my fertility journey.

Life coach and best-selling author Martha Beck, says that many of us find and fulfill our callings by going "to hell and back." She says that once we've been to hell and made it back safely, we often feel called to serve those who are still in hell. That's how I feel. Because I've experienced it myself, I know that infertility can be its own kind of hell, and I hope this book has helped to not only educate you, but offer you comfort. I don't know how I would feel, had I not conceived, however, I know that my spirit would have guided me to exactly where I had to be for the greatest divine good to come of such an experience.

The more I do what I do, the more I love it, and the more awe I feel. And the more we know about fertility, the more I realize, with profound humility, that there is much we don't know. A willingness to be humbled by the mystery of bringing life into the world seems part and parcel of my work as a fertility specialist.

In my desire to bring peace and acceptance to fertility patients everywhere, I am sharing the wisdom in this book as a resource and a stepping stone for your unique and personal journey.

I look forward to hearing your feedback, continuing to offer you new resources, and perhaps, one day, meeting you.

Sincerely, Timea Belej-Rak, M.D.

Contributors

Hoda Abu-Zaid

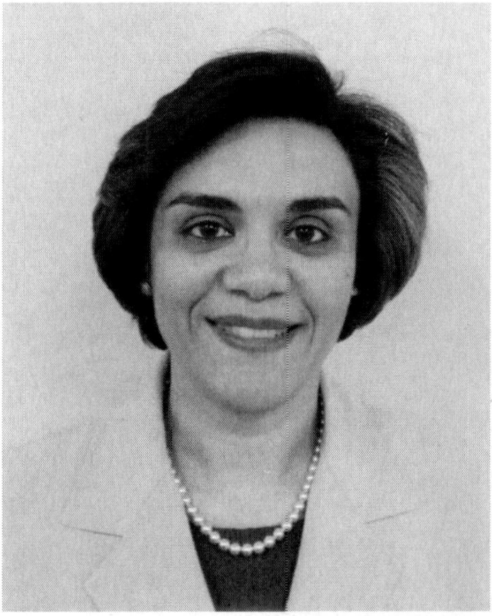

Hoda is a wife and mother of three active young boys, who juggles family and career, while seeking opportunities to grow personally and professionally. She received her honors bachelor of science, and masters of science degrees in nutrition, from the Universities of Toronto and Guelph, respectively. She works corporately within the retail food industry, and is pursuing training through the Institute of Holistic Nutrition to help others achieve optimal health through food and nutrition. An active member of Toastmasters International, Hoda is passionate about public speaking and mentoring others with their speaking skills to help attain their maximum speaking potential.

Haimant Bissessar

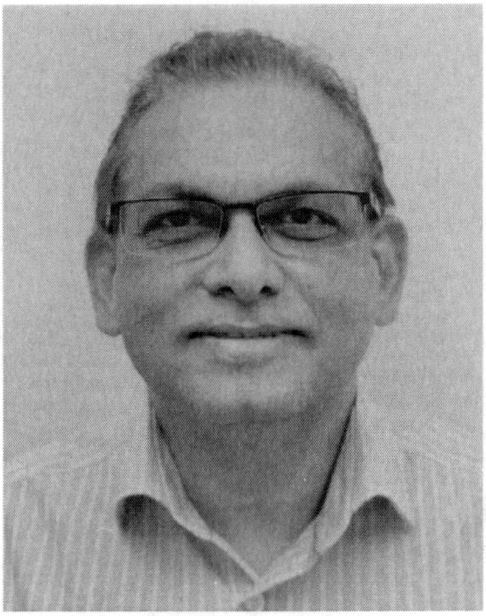

Haimant Bissessar has worked in the field of Assisted Reproductive Technologies (ART) as an embryologist, andrologist and researcher for over thirty years. He received his bachelor of science degree in biology from McMaster University, and his innovative ideas earned him the prestigious Laboratory Innovation in Fertility and Embryology (LIFE) Award. He also co-founded CAN-AM Cryoservices Corp. in 2000, and is its current president. Haimant is an active member of the Canadian Fertility and Andrology Society (CFAS), has a keen interest in ART regulations on donor gamete distribution, and has published many articles on matters of interest to the ART community.

Haimant Bissessar, BSc.

President of CAN-AM Cryoservices Corp.

102-1057 Main Street West, Hamilton, Ontario L8S 1B7

https://www.canamcryo.com/en

hbissessar@canamcryo.com

1-888-245-3471

Glenda Johnson

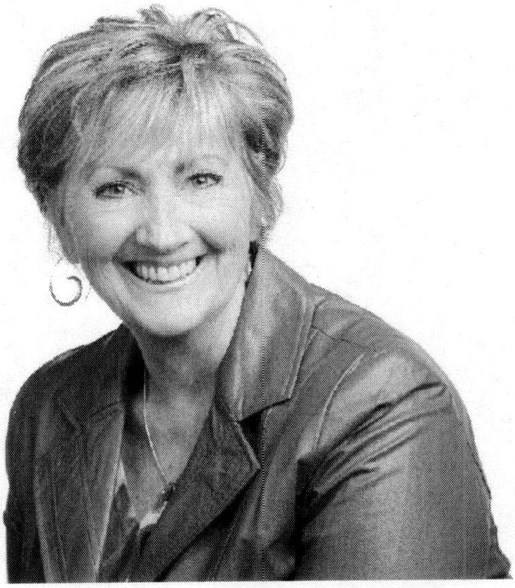

Glenda Johnson is an international relationship coach who is passionate about people, and seeing them succeed where they used to believe it was not possible. Through her tailored approach, she empowers individuals to realize their best life. Glenda believes that everyone can discover, decide on and be successful with their own fertility journey. And that with greater understanding of how life works, they'll begin to be and feel happier because they will re-own their love of self—which is where all self-healing and miracles happen.

Glenda I Johnson, RPT, MCHt

International Relationship Coach

Communication Specialist

www.gijohnson.com

glenda@gijohnsonconsulting.com

905-252-3539

David and Sandra MacDonald

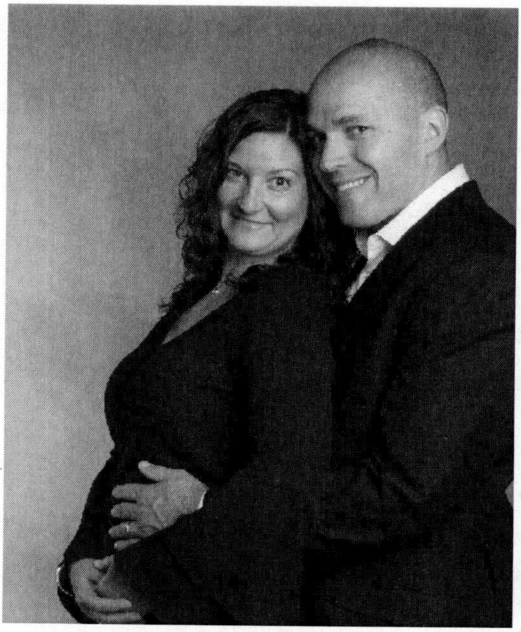

David and Sandra MacDonald are both sales professionals and fitness enthusiasts, who reside just outside Vaughan, Ontario. This couple has experienced the thrill of living and working in Singapore, China and New York City for four-and-a-half of the thirteen years they have been together. Throughout it all, they privately experienced the ups and downs, and heart-wrenching pain of trying to start their own family. Many will have things in common with their story; however, you won't believe the one unique thing that stood in their way of having their first baby.

David Sher

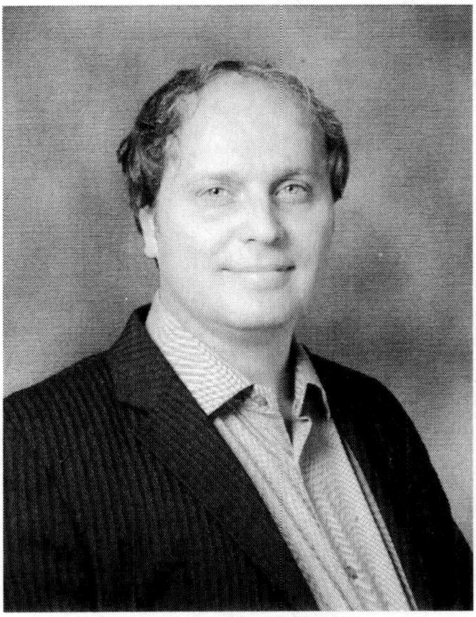

David Sher is the founder, president and CEO of ELITE IVF, a leading global fertility services company established in 2004. He is an expert in cross-border fertility solutions for patients who need IVF treatment using egg donation or surrogacy. During his tenure, ELITE IVF has developed relationships with the world's most renowned fertility clinics resulting in the creation of a first-class medical platform that provides ongoing success to infertility patients from around the world. David Sher has been a pioneer in Canada, transforming ELITE IVF into the first agency in the country to provide egg donation solutions to Canadians abroad.

David Sher, Founder, President, and CEO, ELITE IVF

1 First Canadian Place, Suite 5700 Toronto, ON, M5X 1C7

1 (416) 907-4050, 1 (866) 675-5342

www.elite-ivf.com

david@elite-ivf.com

Sofie Stergianis

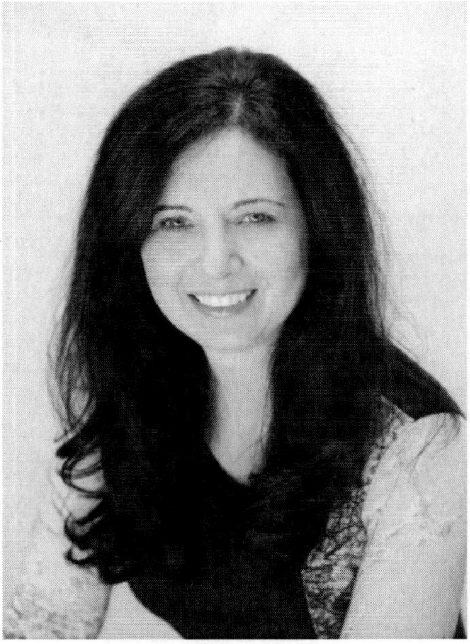

Sofie Stergianis is a private adoption professional who has worked in the field of adoption since 1981. She offers pre- and post-adoption services and counseling to families, and has been instrumental in assisting with the formation of hundreds of adoptive families.

Sofie is also an adoption trainer, who offers a number of education seminars, and has been a keynote speaker at numerous conferences. Sofie is the co-author of the children's book, What is Adoption? Helping Non-Adopted Children Understand Adoption. In her personal life, she is a parent through adoption, and her son, adopted at birth, is now a young adult.

Sofie Stergianis, MSW, RSW

Private Adoption Educator/Practitioner/Co-Author

www.adoptioneducation.ca

Tim H. Tanaka

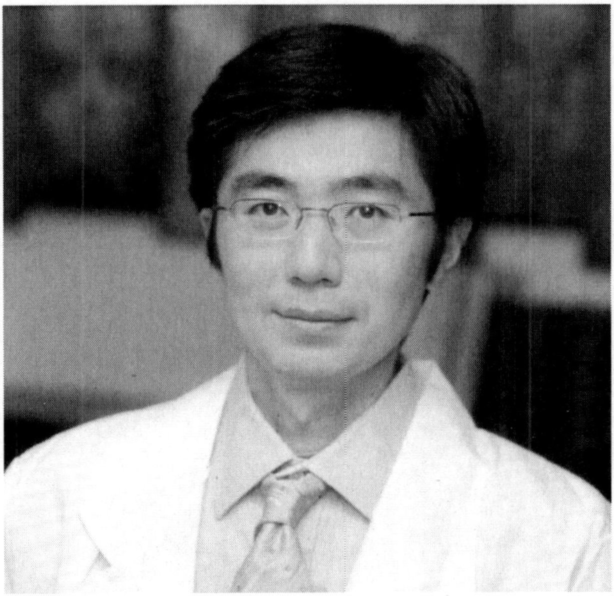

Tim H. Tanaka received his doctor of philosophy degree in medical science in 1996, and is the director of The Pacific Wellness Institute in Toronto. Tim is a nationally licensed acupuncturist in Japan and a registered acupuncturist/Traditional Chinese Medicine practitioner in Ontario. He has co-authored Japanese acupuncture and traditional massage textbooks, in addition to a number of research papers published in peer-reviewed medical journals, and has lectured extensively across the globe. With over thirty years of clinical experience in traditional Asian medicine, Tim has been treating many women using his own unique natural fertility therapy program in his clinic.

Tim H. Tanaka, Ph.D., R.Ac, R.TCMP

Dr. Tanya Wylde

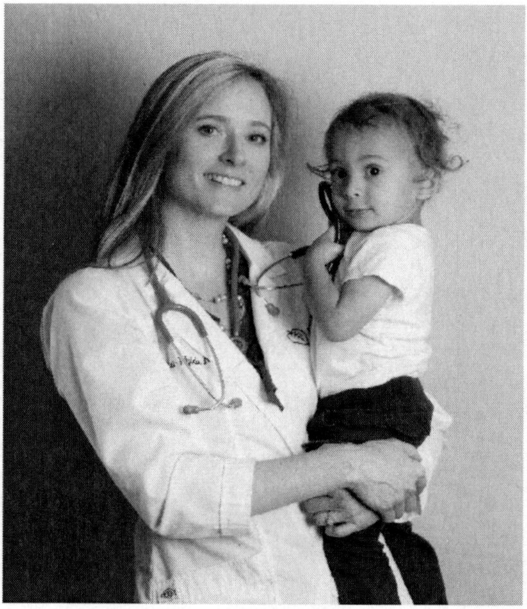

Over the last decade, Dr. Tanya Wylde, a registered naturopathic doctor, has been fortunate to have an extremely busy practice in Vaughan, Ontario, Canada. With an emphasis on therapeutic lifestyle changes, Dr. Wylde has been able to work with thousands of people seeking optimal health. She is committed to health education and empowering her patients with the most current information on health and natural medicine therapies. Tanya has a strong interest in treating fertility issues, hormone imbalances (women's and men's), polycystic ovarian syndrome, weight problems, type 2 diabetes, pregnancy concerns, natural labor, lactation and healthy child development.

Dr. Tanya Wylde, BSc, ND, RAc

Naturopathic Doctor, Registered Acupuncturist

http://wyldenaturalhealthteam.com/about/

https://www.facebook.com/Dr-Tanya-Wylde-Naturopathic-

Doctor-115950228480492/

https://mobile.twitter.com/tanyawylde

https://www.linkedin.com/in/dr-tanya-wylde-nd-b4265475

Reina Zatylny

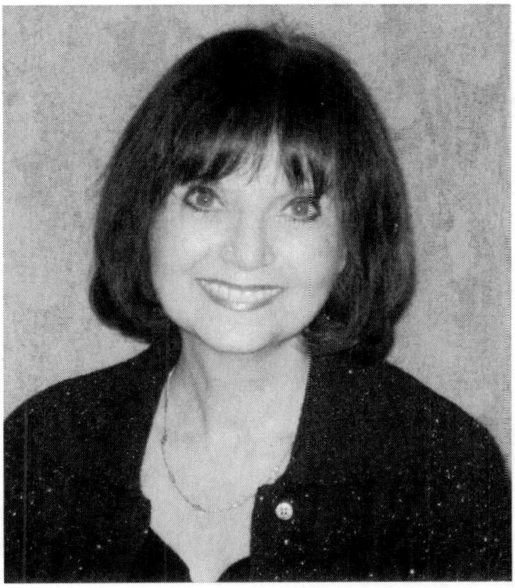

Reina Zatylny, MSW, RSW is a registered clinical social worker and a member of the Ontario College of Social Workers, CFAS, and EMDR Canada. She has a private practice in Toronto, Ontario where she specializes in treating issues involving infertility, relationship discord, trauma, PTSD, addictions, and motor vehicle accidents. Ms. Zatylny is co-chair of the ethics committee at the TRIO fertility clinic, and she is an advisor to and therapist with the Toronto Fire Services. She has developed and conducted seminars for TAPE Educational Services. Her research on couples' relationships has won numerous awards and is published internationally.

Reina Zatylny, MSW, RSW

Individual and Couples Therapist

http://www.reinazatylny.ca/

reina.zatylny@sympatico.ca

416-540-5924

About the Author

Timea Belej-Rak

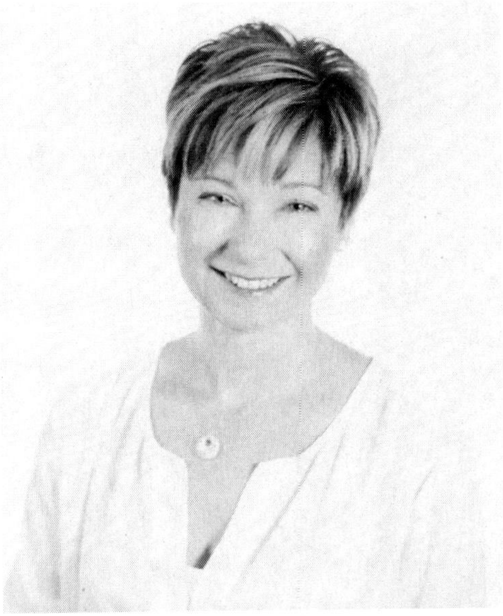

Your fertility is Dr. Timea's number one priority because she understands how stressful your journey can be. She has been a practicing fertility specialist for the past fifteen years, and believes in a healing and prevention-based approach to health and well-being, supported by ongoing education and research. This system, which takes into account the whole person (body, mind, and spirit) and their environment, uses a wide range of complementary and conventional therapies. Dr. Timea uses all of these tools to provide individualized patient care with you as her focus.

Timea Belej-Rak, BSc, MSc, MD, FRCSC, GREI

Belej-Rak Medicine Professional Corporation

FemWellness - Integrative Women's Health & Fertility

Gynecologic Reproductive Endocrinology & Infertility

191 McNaughton Road East, Suite 401

Timea Belej-Rak, M.D.

Maple, Ontario, L6A 4E2

T: 289-553-0216 ext. 221

F: 1-833-217-9884

www.femwellness.ca

https://www.facebook.com/YourFertilityCanada

www.twitter.com/tbelejrak

https://ca.linkedin.com/pub/timea-belej-rak/1a/b19/295

Made in United States
Cleveland, OH
06 November 2026

47781106R00108